Hospitalized Chronic Pain Patient

David A. Edwards · Padma Gulur
Christopher M. Sobey
Editors

Hospitalized Chronic Pain Patient

A Multidisciplinary Treatment Guide

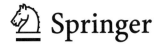 Springer

Editors
David A. Edwards
Departments of Anesthesiology and
Neurological Surgery
Vanderbilt University Medical Center
Nashville, TN, USA

Padma Gulur
Department of Anesthesiology
Duke University Health System
Durham, NC, USA

Christopher M. Sobey
Department of Anesthesiology
Vanderbilt University Medical Center
Nashville, TN, USA

ISBN 978-3-031-08378-5   ISBN 978-3-031-08376-1   (eBook)
https://doi.org/10.1007/978-3-031-08376-1

This Springer imprint is published by the registered company Springer Nature Switzerland AG
The registered company address is: Gewerbestrasse 11, 6330 Cham, Switzerland

Preface

Hospitalized Chronic Pain Patient is a text intended to improve the care of patients with chronic pain admitted to the hospital either because of pain or with other health conditions. These patients are at risk of suffering due to under- or even overtreatment, leading to adverse outcomes.

The material in this text will assist the learner, the teacher, and the life-long learning practitioner by providing basic considerations for treating acute and chronic pain in the hospital. The text may also serve as a quick reference, review manual, or teaching tool for teachers on rounds.

Management of chronic pain patients can be quite challenging at baseline and often significantly more so during acute exacerbations while inpatient. Best in class care would ensure communication at admission or preoperatively if an elective surgical admission, with the patient's chronic care provider to establish baseline needs as highlighted in this text. The materials further cover evidence-based approaches to inpatient management and a clear pathway to transitional support as the patient is discharged to ensure a smooth return to baseline and optimal outcomes.

We hope this handbook provides guidance in management decisions to facilitate expeditious, effective, and compassionate care.

We acknowledge the long list of skilled authors and their expertise succinctly summarized in the chapters herein. We are grateful to our mentors who have taught us: Dr. Andre Boezaart for his mentorship and singular focus on doing the right thing, for the right patient, for the right reason; Dr. Marc Huntoon for his guidance in clinical judgment and incorporating innovative strategies in the treatment algorithm when appropriate; Dr. Jianren Mao for providing and teaching us the underlying mechanisms of pain that direct a mechanistic and more effective approach to treatment. We would like to thank the Springer staff for their assistance and direction. Last, but not least, we would like to thank our families and friends for their love and support while pursuing this project.

We hope this treatment guide provides those who read it the tools to achieve our goal of advancing excellent patient care and improving clinical outcomes for a vulnerable patient population. We strive to improve access to and quality of care for our patients while in the hospital and following discharge.

Nashville, TN, USA David A. Edwards
Durham, NC, USA Padma Gulur
Nashville, TN, USA Christopher M. Sobey

Contents

Part III   Cases

Part VI   Palliative Care

Part VII   Discharge

Contributors

Meredith C. B. Adams, M.D., M.S. Department of Anesthesiology, Wake Forest Baptist Health, Winston-Salem, NC, USA

Brian F. S. Allen, M.D. Department of Anesthesiology, Vanderbilt University Medical Center, Nashville, TN, USA

Vikram Bansal, M.D. Department of Anesthesiology, Vanderbilt University Medical Center, Nashville, TN, USA

Thomas E. Buchheit, M.D. Department of Anesthesiology, Duke University School of Medicine, Durham, NC, USA

David Byrne, M.D. U.S. Anesthesia Partners, Dallas, TX, USA

Greg Carpenter, M.D., M.B.A. Department of Anesthesiology, VA Tennessee Valley Healthcare System, Nashville, TN, USA

C. Terrell Cummings, M.D. Momentum Spine and Joint, Arlington, TX, USA

Bethany-Rose Daubman, M.D. Division of Palliative Care and Geriatrics, Department of Medicine, Massachusetts General Hospital, Harvard University, Boston, MA, USA

Rakhi Dayal, M.D. Department of Anesthesiology, University of California, Irvine, Orange, CA, USA

Rebecca Donald, M.D. Department of Anesthesiology, Vanderbilt University Medical Center, Nashville, TN, USA

Daltry Dott, M.D. Department of Anesthesiology, University of Texas Southwestern, Dallas, TX, USA

David A. Edwards, M.D. Ph.D. Departments of Anesthesiology and Neurological Surgery, Vanderbilt University Medical Center, Nashville, TN, USA

Arun Ganesh, M.D. Department of Anesthesiology, Duke University School of Medicine, Durham, NC, USA

Jeff A. Gartner, M.D. Department of Anesthesiology, Ascension Medical Group, Nashville, TN, USA

Peter V. Gikas, M.D. Aurora Health Care, Milwaukee, WI, USA

Brandon Gish, M.D. Commonwealth Pain and Spine, Nicholasville, KY, USA
Commonwealth Pain and Spine, Lexington, KY, USA

Burel R. Goodin, Ph.D. Department of Psychology, University of Alabama at Birmingham, Birmingham, AL, USA
Department of Anesthesiology and Perioperative Medicine, University of Alabama at Birmingham, Birmingham, AL, USA

Padma Gulur, M.D. Department of Anesthesiology, Duke University Health System, Durham, NC, USA

Ginger E. Holt, M.D. Department of Orthopaedics, Vanderbilt University Medical Center, Nashville, TN, USA

Christopher Howson, M.D. BayCare Clinic Pain and Rehab Medicine, Green Bay, WI, USA

Tracy P. Jackson, M.D. Bright Heart Health, Walnut Creek, CA, USA

Maxwell James, M.D. Department of Anesthesiology, Vanderbilt University Medical Center, Nashville, TN, USA

Mihir M. Kamdar, M.D. Division of Palliative Care, Massachusetts General Hospital, Harvard University, Boston, MA, USA
Division of Anesthesia Pain Medicine, Massachusetts General Hospital, Harvard University, Boston, MA, USA

Michael Kent, M.D. Department of Anesthesiology, Duke University Health System, Durham, NC, USA

Gwynne Kirchen, M.D. Medical College of Wisconsin, Milwaukee, WI, USA

Shaun Kuoni, M.D. The NeuroMedical Center Clinic, Hammond, LA, USA

Katheryne Lawson, M.D. Department of Anesthesiology, Royal Children's Hospital Melbourne, Parkville, VIC, Australia

Eugene Leytin, M.D. Bend Anesthesiology Group, Bend, OR, USA

Daniel Lonergan, M.D. Cuyuna Regional Medical Center, Crosby, MN, USA

Benjamin J. MacDougall, M.D. Department of Anesthesiology, Vanderbilt University Medical Center, Nashville, TN, USA

David Marcovitz, M.D. Department of Psychiatry, Vanderbilt University Medical Center, Nashville, TN, USA

Melissa McKittrick, M.D. Department of Anesthesiology, Vanderbilt University Medical Center, Nashville, TN, USA

Puneet Mishra, M.D. Department of Anesthesiology, Vanderbilt University Medical Center, Nashville, TN, USA

Melisa Z. Murphy, M.D. North Texas Orthopedics and Spine Center, Grapevine, TX, USA

Hai Nguyen, D.O. Minivasive Pain and Orthopedics, Spring, TX, USA

Obi Okwuchukwu, M.D. Las Vegas Pain Institute, Las Vegas, NV, USA

Atish Patel, M.D. Department of Anesthesiology, Northwestern Medical Center, Chicago, IL, USA

Andrew J. B. Pisansky, M.D., M.S. Department of Anesthesiology, Vanderbilt University Medical Center, Nashville, TN, USA

Lauren Poe, D.O. Department of Anesthesiology, Vanderbilt University Medical Center, Nashville, TN, USA

Myrick C. Shinall Jr, M.D., Ph.D. Department of Surgery, Vanderbilt University Medical Center, Nashville, TN, USA

Christopher M. Sobey, M.D. Department of Anesthesiology, Vanderbilt University Medical Center, Nashville, TN, USA

Stacy D. Tillman, M.D. Department of Medicine, Division of Palliative Care, Vanderbilt University Medical Center, Nashville, TN, USA

Stephanie G. Vanterpool, M.D., M.B.A., F.A.S.A. Department of Anesthesiology, University of Tennessee Graduate School of Medicine, Knoxville, TN, USA

Jenna L. Walters, M.D. Midlands Orthopaedics and Neurosurgery, Columbia, SC, USA

Katherine Williams, M.D. Commonwealth Pain and Spine, Evansville, IN, USA

Robert J. Wilson II, M.D. Department of Orthopaedics, Baptist MD Anderson Cancer Center, Jacksonville, FL, USA

Kristen M. Woods, M.A. Department of Medicine, University of Alabama at Birmingham, Birmingham, AL, USA

Andrew Wooldridge, M.D. Department of Medicine, Division of Palliative Care, Vanderbilt University Medical Center, Nashville, TN, USA

April Zehm, M.D., F.A.A.H.P.M. Division of Geriatric and Palliative Medicine, Clinical Cancer Center, Medical College of Wisconsin, Milwaukee, WI, USA

Abbreviations

AIDS	Acquired immunodeficiency syndrome
ASRA	American Society of Regional Anesthesia and Pain Medicine
BID	*Bis in die* (twice a day)
BKP	Balloon kyphoplasty
BPI	Brief pain inventory
BTX	Botulinum toxin
cAMP	Cyclic adenosine monophosphate
CB	Cannabinoid receptor (CB1, CB2)
CBD	Cannabidiol
CBT	Cognitive behavioral therapy
CGRP	Calcitonin gene-related peptide
CKD	Chronic kidney disease
COPD	Chronic obstructive pulmonary disease
COWS	Clinical opiate withdrawal scale
CrCl	Creatinine clearance
CRP	C-reactive protein
CRPS	Chronic regional pain syndrome
CSF	Cerebral spinal fluid
CT	Computed tomography
DDD	Drug delivery device
DNA	Deoxyribonucleic acid
DREZ	Dorsal root entry zone
DVPRS	Defense and veterans pain rating scale
ECG	Electrocardiogram
ED	Emergency department
EMS	Emergency medical services
ESR	Erythrocyte sedimentation rate
FABER	Flexion, abduction, external rotation (Patrick's test)
FLACC	Face, legs, activity, cry, consolability scale
GABA	Gamma-aminobutyric acid
HIV	Human immunodeficiency virus
IT	Intrathecal

ITB	Intrathecal baclofen
LA	Local anesthetic
LAST	Local anesthetic systemic toxicity
LE	Law enforcement
MAT	Medication for addiction treatment, or medication-assisted treatment
MCA	Middle cerebral artery
MEDD	Morphine equivalent daily dose
MMA	Multimodal analgesia
MME	Milligram morphine equivalent
MOA	Mechanism of action
MRI	Magnetic resonance imaging
MS	Multiple sclerosis
NAS	Neonatal abstinence syndrome
NMDA	*N*-methyl-D-aspartate
NOWS	Neonatal opioid withdrawal syndrome
NSAID	Nonsteroidal anti-inflammatory drug
OA	Osteoarthritis
OIC	Opioid-induced constipation
OIH	Opioid-induced hyperalgesia
ORT	Opioid risk tool
OSA	Obstructive sleep apnea
OUD	Opioid use disorder
PCA	Patient-controlled analgesia
PDPH	Postdural puncture headache
PET	Positron emission tomography
PRN	*Pro re nata* (as needed)
PRO	Patient-reported outcome
PVP	Percutaneous vertebroplasty
QID	*Quater in die* (four times a day)
QoR	Quality of recovery
QST	Quantitative sensory testing
RA	Rheumatoid arthritis
SBIRT	Screening, brief intervention, referral to treatment
SCD	Sickle cell disease
SCRIPT	Story, current symptoms, Rx (relevant medications), interventions, physical therapy, tests
SCS	Spinal cord stimulation
SNRI	Serotonin norepinephrine reuptake inhibitor
SSRI	Selective serotonin reuptake inhibitor
STIR	Short tau inversion recovery MRI image
SUD	Substance use disorder
TCA	Tricyclic antidepressant
TENS	Transcutaneous electrical nerve stimulation

THC	Tetrahydrocannabinol
TID	*Ter in die* (three times a day)
TRPV1	Transient receptor potential cation channel subtype 1
UMN	Upper motor neuron
VAS	Visual analogue scale
VCF	Vertebral compression fracture
VGSC	Voltage-gated sodium channel

Introduction to the Chronic Pain Patient

David A. Edwards and Padma Gulur

Introduction

There are over 50 million people living with chronic pain in the United States [1]. Nearly 20 million have high impact chronic pain and live each day either succeeding or failing in their attempt to manage it and live functional lives [1]. When patients with chronic pain are hospitalized they often feel anxiety and fear not only about their acute illness but also about how pain will be managed. Often they are undertreated and suffer, are at increased risk for morbidity and mortality, stay longer in the hospital, are readmitted earlier and more frequently, are dissatisfied with their care, and rate hospitals poorly [2–7].

On behalf of patients with chronic pain, we gathered practical treatment information into this new manual so more learners understand that there are more options for controlling pain in hospitalized patients. In fact, each new day brings advances in medical knowledge about pain mechanisms and treatment options. Learners need to be aware of these options to provide targeted treatment at the lowest risk to patients. Targeted treatment is specific to the mechanism underlying the type of pain and is thereby more effective. Targeted treatment of pain may prevent future complications such as worsened chronic pain or the development of opioid use disorder.

The *Hospitalized Chronic Pain Patient* manual was developed to be used, not just read. The authors are educators at institutions with highly regarded acute pain, chronic pain, palliative care, and surgical programs. Each chapter is short and full

D. A. Edwards (✉)
Departments of Anesthesiology and Neurological Surgery, Vanderbilt University Medical Center, Nashville, TN, USA
e-mail: david.a.edwards@vumc.org

P. Gulur
Department of Anesthesiology, Duke University Health System, Durham, NC, USA
e-mail: padma.gulur@duke.edu

© Springer Nature Switzerland AG 2022
D. A. Edwards et al. (eds.), *Hospitalized Chronic Pain Patient*,
https://doi.org/10.1007/978-3-031-08376-1_1

of summary bullet points and tables for quick reference and teaching during rounds. The manual starts by introducing key concepts and terms when discussing and measuring pain. Seventeen case examples provide relevant considerations and information for the management of chronic pain in patients admitted to the hospital. Medical, interventional, surgical, and palliative care treatment options are then presented. Finally, the manual ends with a section outlining transition plans for hospital discharge, de-escalation of acute care and the resumption of outpatient chronic pain management.

We dedicate this manual to patients and hope that the shortcomings in our knowledge about the mechanisms and best treatments for pain will soon be overcome.

References

1. Dahlhamer J, Lucas J, Zelaya C, et al. Prevalence of chronic pain and high-impact chronic pain among adults—United States, 2016. MMWR Morb Mortal Wkly Rep. 2018;67(36):1001–6.
2. Brennan F, Carr DB, Cousins M. Pain management: a fundamental human right. Anesth Analg. 2007;105(1):205–21.
3. Albrecht E, Taffe P, Yersin B, et al. Undertreatment of acute pain (oligoanalgesia) and medical practice variation in prehospital analgesia of adult trauma patients: a 10 year retrospective study. Br J Anaesth. 2013;110(1):96–106.
4. Gulur P, Williams L, Chaudhary S, et al. Opioid tolerance—a predictor of increased length of stay and higher readmission rates. Pain Physician. 2014;17(4):E503–7.
5. Cole BE. Pain management: classifying, understanding, and treating pain. Hosp Physician. 2002;2002:14991685.
6. Herzig SJ, Rothberg MB, Cheung M, et al. Opioid utilization and opioid-related adverse events in nonsurgical patients in US hospitals. J Hosp Med. 2014;9(2):73–81.
7. Apfelbaum JL, Chen C, Mehta SS, Gan TJ. Postoperative pain experience: results from a national survey suggest postoperative pain continues to be undermanaged. Anesth Analg. 2003;97(2):534–40.

Definitions

2

David A. Edwards and Puneet Mishra

Introduction

Listed alphabetically are several key terms that are important to understand when discussing the concept of pain [1]. Many other important terms are included within the relevant chapters.

Allodynia—Pain elicited from typically non-painful stimuli.

Analgesia—Relief or absence of, lessening or insensibility to pain.

Anesthesia—Loss of sensation.

Dolorosa—A painful sensation. For example, anesthesia dolorosa is a painful sensation in an area that is numb or with loss of sensation.

Dysesthesia—Abnormal or impaired sensation.

Hyperaesthesia—Abnormal increased sensation to stimuli.

Hyperalgesia—Abnormal increased sensation to painful stimuli.

Hypoesthesia—Abnormal decreased sensation to stimuli.

Neuralgia—Nerve related pain.

Neuritis—Inflammation of a nerve often causing pain.

Neuropathy—Disease or damage causing dysfunction of a nerve.

Noxious—Causing or potentially causing damage.

Nociception—The neural detection and processing of noxious stimuli.

D. A. Edwards
Departments of Anesthesiology and Neurological Surgery, Vanderbilt University Medical Center, Nashville, TN, USA
e-mail: david.a.edwards@vumc.org

P. Mishra (✉)
Department of Anesthesiology, Vanderbilt University Medical Center, Nashville, TN, USA
e-mail: puneet.mishra@vumc.org

© Springer Nature Switzerland AG 2022
D. A. Edwards et al. (eds.), *Hospitalized Chronic Pain Patient*,
https://doi.org/10.1007/978-3-031-08376-1_2

Nociplastic pain—Pain from disordered nociception in the absence of a noxious stimulus.

Pain—A personal sensory and emotional response associated with noxious stimuli.

Paresthesia—Abnormal sensation.

Reference

1. Merskey H, Bogduk N. Part III: Pain terms: a current list with definitions and notes on usage. In: Classification of chronic pain. 2nd ed. Washington, DC: IASP Task Force on Taxonomy; 1994. p. 209–14.

Part I

Pathophysiology

Acute Pain

3

David A. Edwards and Puneet Mishra

Relationship of Acute Pain to Chronic Pain

Pain can be classified temporally (Fig. 3.1). John Bonica originally described and defined acute pain in 1953 and differentiated it from chronic pain as pain that persists beyond the usual course of tissue healing [1]. Harold Merskey and Nikolai Bogduk categorized acute pain as generally being <3 months and chronic pain >3 months [2, 3]. More recently, the concept of subacute pain as an extension of the acute pain period has been described that may involve underlying processes in transition to chronic pain [4].

Acute pain can be further classified qualitatively, by pain type (Table 3.1) taking a mechanistic approach that helps guide targeted treatment (see also Chap. 7) [5].

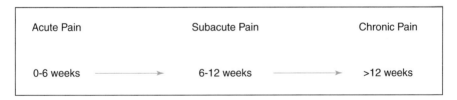

Acute Pain	Subacute Pain	Chronic Pain
0-6 weeks	6-12 weeks	>12 weeks

Fig. 3.1 Acute, subacute, and chronic pain

D. A. Edwards
Departments of Anesthesiology and Neurological Surgery, Vanderbilt University Medical Center, Nashville, TN, USA
e-mail: david.a.edwards@vumc.org

P. Mishra (✉)
Department of Anesthesiology, Vanderbilt University Medical Center, Nashville, TN, USA
e-mail: puneet.mishra@vumc.org

© Springer Nature Switzerland AG 2022
D. A. Edwards et al. (eds.), *Hospitalized Chronic Pain Patient*,
https://doi.org/10.1007/978-3-031-08376-1_3

Table 3.1 Classification of pain type

Somatic nociceptive pain	Inflammatory pain	Neuropathic pain
• Musculoskeletal (fracture, wounds)	• Inflammatory mediators directly activate neurons (infection, arthritis)	• Diabetic or chemotherapy-induced neuropathy
Visceral nociceptive pain		Central and dysfunctional pain
• Organs (stomach, pancreas, bowel)		• Acute sensitization (regional hyperalgesia), chronic sensitization (fibromyalgia)

Table 3.2 Nerve fiber types

Large fiber (fast)	Aα myelinated (motor, proprioception)
	Aβ myelinated (touch, pressure)
	Aγ myelinated (proprioception)
Medium fiber (moderate-fast)	Aδ thinly myelinated (cold temperature, heat pain, pressure pain)
	B thinly myelinated (autonomic, sympathetic)
Small fiber (slow)	C unmyelinated (heat, heat pain, pressure pain, sympathetic)

Mechanism of Acute Pain

Pain is transmitted from the peripheral nervous system structures to the central nervous system where it is perceived. Peripheral structures that detect and transmit pain include several different nerve fiber types, pain receptors and nerve free endings (Table 3.2).

Treatment of Acute Pain

The severity of acute pain has a strong association with the development of chronic pain [6]. Therefore, treatment of severe acute pain in a timely fashion is important. Treatment is most effective when the therapy is targeted to the pain type (Table 3.1). Firstly, acute pain may be a sign of disease, and treatment of the disease should be the primary focus. Secondly, pain relief can be sufficiently attained through effective non-medication therapies such as through movement, such as with guided physical therapy. Medication and procedural interventions can be effective adjuncts to palliate the severity of acute pain and enable recovery (Table 3.3).

Table 3.3 Pain therapies

Non-medication pain therapies	Medication pain therapies
Mechanical treatments	Nociceptive pain
• Braces, splints	• Muscle relaxers (methocarbamol, cyclobenzaprine, tizanidine, baclofen)
• Heat, cold	• Acetaminophen
• Physical therapy, occupational therapy, aquatherapy, lymphedema therapy, desensitization therapy, mirror therapy	• Opioids
• Needling, acupuncture	Inflammatory pain
• Massage	• NSAIDs (ibuprofen, ketorolac, naproxen, meloxicam)
• Transcutaneous electrical nerve stimulation (TENS)	• Steroids (prednisone, methylprednisolone)
• Chiropractic treatment	Central and dysfunctional pain
Psychology	• Anticonvulsants (gabapentin, pregabalin)
• Cognitive behavioral therapy (CBT)	• Serotonin–norepinephrine reuptake inhibitors (SNRIs) (duloxetine, venlafaxine, milnacipran)
• Biofeedback	• Tricyclic anti-depressants (TCAs) (nortriptyline, amitriptyline, desipramine)
• Mindfulness	• Na^+ channel blockers (lidocaine, mexiletine, topiramate, carbamazepine)
• Hypnosis	• TRPV1 ion channel (capsaicin)
	• NMDA antagonists (ketamine, memantine)

References

1. Bonica JJ. The management of pain. Philadelphia: Lea & Febiger; 1953.
2. Merskey H. Pain terms: a list with definitions and notes on usage recommended by the IASP Subcommittee on Taxonomy. Pain. 1979;6:249–52.
3. Merskey H, Bogduk N. Classification of chronic pain. Descriptions of chronic pain syndromes and definitions of pain terms. 2nd ed. Seattle: IASP Press; 1994. p. 9.
4. van Tulder MW, Koes BW, Bouter LM. Conservative treatment of acute and chronic nonspecific low back pain. A systematic review of randomized controlled trials of the most common interventions. Spine. 1997;22:2128–56.
5. Vardeh D, Mannion RJ, Woolf CJ. Toward a mechanism-based approach to pain diagnosis. J Pain. 2016;17(9 Suppl):T50–69.
6. Puolakka P, Rorarius M, Roviola M, Puolakka T, Nordhausen K, Lindgren L. Persistent pain following knee arthroplasty. Eur J Anaesthesiol. 2010;27(5):455–60.

Chronic Pain

Melisa Z. Murphy, Tracy P. Jackson, and Puneet Mishra

4

Prevalence and Risk Factors

Over 50 million people in the United States live with chronic pain, and over 19 million have high impact chronic pain requiring ongoing treatment [1, 2] (Fig. 4.1). The following tables show the prevalence of chronic pain in post-surgical conditions (Table 4.1) [3, 4], and the common risk factors associated with the development of chronic post-surgical pain (Table 4.2) [5].

Pathophysiology of Chronic Pain

Phase I: Acute Surgical Response and Acute Pain

During surgery or initial cellular injury, inflammatory mediators are activated to cause localized pain.

Pro-inflammatory mediators include hydrogen, potassium ions, bradykinin, prostaglandins, and cytokines (IL-2, IL-6, IL-8 and TNF-alpha) [6, 7]. After the stimulus is gone and inflammatory mediators subside, nociceptive receptor sensitivity should return to normal. However, persistent receptor hypersensitivity indicates central sensitization.

M. Z. Murphy
North Texas Orthopedics and Spine Center, Grapevine, TX, USA

T. P. Jackson
Bright Heart Health, Walnut Creek, CA, USA

P. Mishra (✉)
Department of Anesthesiology, Vanderbilt University Medical Center, Nashville, TN, USA
e-mail: puneet.mishra@vumc.org

© Springer Nature Switzerland AG 2022
D. A. Edwards et al. (eds.), *Hospitalized Chronic Pain Patient*,
https://doi.org/10.1007/978-3-031-08376-1_4

11

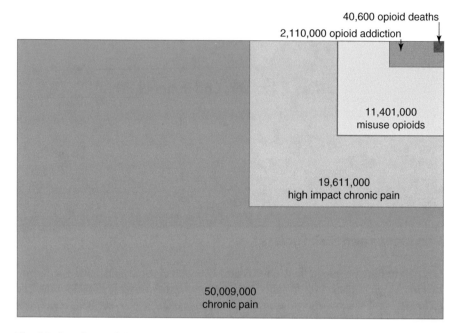

Fig. 4.1 Prevalence of chronic pain and opioid addiction in the United States

Table 4.1 Prevalence of chronic post-surgical pain

Surgical types	Prevalence (%)
Hernia repair	13.6
Vaginal hysterectomy	11.8
Mastectomy	13–69
Thoracotomy	37.6
Video-assisted thoracic surgery	25
Amputation (including phantom pain)	67
Lung transplant	5–10
Total knee replacement	10
Total hip replacement	20

Table 4.2 Risk factors for chronic post-surgical pain

Surgical factors	Direct neural trauma: amputation, thoracotomy
Anesthesia factors	Severe uncontrolled postop pain
Patient factors	Age
	Physical health via short form health survey
	Mental health survey
	Preoperative pain in the surgical field
	Preoperative pain in other areas
	Female
	Depression
	Post-traumatic stress disorder
	Anxiety
	Hypervigilant state towards surgery

Phase II: Centralized Chronic Pain

Central sensitization is an increased responsiveness of neurocircuitry in the central nervous system to noxious stimuli. The increased responsiveness may be due enhanced neuronal function and signal transmission that results in facilitated action potential output [8]. Underlying processes may be due to modulation (reversible) or modification (potentially irreversible) in neuronal structures and include changes in brain activity, synaptic efficacy (e.g., neuroplastic changes, lowering of pain stimulus threshold), receptor field expansion [8]. The reversible modulations caused by acute pain stimuli may become irreversible with repetitive stimulation.

Prevention and Treatment Principles of Chronic Pain

Modifiable risk factors associated with chronic pain represent potential avenues for treatment that may reduce the likelihood that acute pain becomes chronic. However, to date, pre-surgical pre-emptive techniques have yet to show significant success at reduction of the development of prolonged post-surgical pain. What has been successful is targeting the disease process itself, thereby preventing severe disease and development of severe chronic pain (e.g., controlled diabetes). Given the strong association the severity of acute pain has with the development of chronic pain, interventional techniques like the use of ketamine infusions or regional anesthesia may eventually demonstrate a reduction in the development of chronic pain [9, 10].

Conclusion

There has been increased interest in understanding the significance and pathophysiology of acute pain becoming chronic. Identifying patients at risk of developing chronic pain, understanding the mechanism, and employing multimodal therapy for pain management can help to reduce the prevalence of chronic pain, decrease healthcare cost and improve public health.

References

1. Dahlhamer J, et al. Prevalence of chronic pain and high-impact chronic pain among adults—United States, 2016. MMWR Morb Mortal Wkly Rep. 2018;67(36):1001–6.
2. Substance Abuse and Mental Health Services Administration. Results from the 2018 National Survey on Drug Use and Health: detailed tables. Rockville: Substance Abuse and Mental Health Services Administration; 2019.
3. Neil MJE, Bannister J. When acute pain becomes chronic. Anaesthesia. 2015;70:779–83.
4. Macrae WA. Chronic post-surgical pain: 10 years on. Br J Anaesth. 2008;101:77–86.
5. Perkins FM, Kehlet H. Chronic pain as an outcome of surgery. A review of predictive factors. Anesthesiology. 2000;93(4):1123–33.

6. Kehlet H, Jensen TS, Woolf CJ. Persistent postsurgical pain: risk factors and prevention. Lancet. 2006;367:1618–25.
7. Voscopoulos C, Lema M. When does acute pain becomes chronic. Br J Anaesth. 2010; 105(suppl 1):i69–85.
8. Woolf CJ. Central sensitization: implications for the diagnosis and treatment of pain. Pain. 2011;152(Suppl P):S2–S15.
9. Jahangiri M, Jayatunga AP, Bradley JW, Dark CH. Prevention of phantom pain after major lower limb amputation by epidural infusion of diamorphine, clonidine and bupivacaine. Ann R Coll Surg Engl. 1994;76(5):324–6.
10. Gupta A, Gandhi K, Viscusi ER. Persistent postsurgical pain after abdominal surgery. Tech Reg Anesth Pain Manag. 2011;15(3):140–6.

Opioid-Induced Hyperalgesia

5

Melisa Z. Murphy, David A. Edwards, and Puneet Mishra

Clinical Examples of OIH

Two common clinical scenarios where patient may experience OIH are (1) following remifentanil infusion in the immediate postoperative period and (2) in chronic methadone users. In 2014, two systematic reviews were published about OIH by intraoperative remifentanil use [1, 2]. Both groups recognized that in many situations the clinical relevance was questionable.

Remifentanil

In the operating room, remifentanil used to treat operative pain is advantageous due to its rapid metabolism by plasma and tissue esterases. The context sensitive half-time is 4 min. If no other analgesia is provided, patients may experience hyperalgesia after being treated with remifentanil. This is often measured by demonstrating that patients treated with remifentanil require more postoperative opioids [1, 2]. Several trials systematically reviewed using ketamine, nitrous, magnesium, clonidine, pregabalin, dexmedetomidine show inconsistent evidence preventing remifentanil-induced hyperalgesia.

M. Z. Murphy
North Texas Orthopedics and Spine Center, Grapevine, TX, USA

D. A. Edwards (✉)
Departments of Anesthesiology and Neurological Surgery, Vanderbilt University Medical Center, Nashville, TN, USA
e-mail: david.a.edwards@vumc.org

P. Mishra
Department of Anesthesiology, Vanderbilt University Medical Center, Nashville, TN, USA
e-mail: puneet.mishra@vumc.org

© Springer Nature Switzerland AG 2022
D. A. Edwards et al. (eds.), *Hospitalized Chronic Pain Patient*,
https://doi.org/10.1007/978-3-031-08376-1_5

Methadone

Among studies in chronic methadone users, 11 out of 13 clinical trials showed lower threshold to cold pain. There were mixed results with electrical pain or heat pain stimulation [3].

Mechanism Underlying OIH

Opioid receptors concentrate in peripheral nociceptive fibers that synapse centrally upon spinal dorsal horn neurons, and in pathways descending from the rostral ventral medial medulla to the spinal cord [4, 5]. Under normal conditions, when exogenous opioids activate opioid receptors, a cascade of changes in downstream second messenger systems leads to decreased neuronal transmission of pain.

The mechanism for opioid analgesia has been clearly delineated over the past several decades. Opioid receptors belong to the class of seven-transmembrane domain G-protein coupled inhibitory receptors. When ligands bind, the receptors activate Gi/o which dissociates into α and $\beta\gamma$ subunits [6]. Gi/o inhibits adenylyl cyclase (AC) activity, downstream levels of cyclic adenosine monophosphate (cAMP) are reduced, and protein kinase activity is reduced (Fig. 5.1a). Potassium channels are made more permeable while calcium channels become less permeable, causing presynaptic terminals to hyperpolarize, decreasing the release of glutamate and substance P [4]. Postsynaptic terminals are also hyperpolarized resulting in decreased neuronal excitability and reduced signal transduction [5]. With respect to

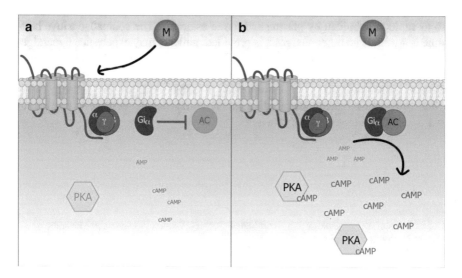

Fig. 5.1 (**a**) Morphine (M) activates the 7-transmembrane opioid receptor coupled to Gi, that inhibits adenylyl cyclase (AC). (**b**) In AC superactivation, even after morphine no longer acts on the opioid receptor, AC remains active, cAMP levels are increased, and PKA is active

pain signal sensitivity and transmission of nociceptive signals, the neuronal cell becomes quiescent with acute opioid receptor binding.

After chronic opioid exposure, however, in vitro studies show the situation is nearly reversed (Fig. 5.1b). Chronic opioid activation of μ-, and δ-opioid receptors transfected into neuronal cell types leads to Raf-1 mediated phosphorylation of AC [7]. Raf-1 phosphorylation of AC increases its activity, 24 a process called AC superactivation [8]. This leads to increased cAMP production and augmentation of protein kinase A (PKA), which in turn enhances increases the release of pain enhancing neurotransmitters such as calcitonin gene-related peptide (CGRP). Morphine also sensitizes AC toward Gs protein-coupled excitatory transmitters such as PGE2, which is released with tissue injury. This also causes release of the pain enhancing neurotransmitter CGRP. AC superactivation by sustained opioid administration therefore appears to be one likely contributor to OIH.

References

1. Martinez V, Fletcher D. Prevention of opioid-induced hyperalgesia in surgical patients: does it really matter? Br J Anaesth. 2012;109:302–4.
2. Rivosecchi RM, Rice MJ, Smithburger PL, et al. An evidence based systematic review of remifentanil associated opioid-induced hyperalgesia. Expert Opin Drug Saf. 2014;13:587–603.
3. Edwards DA, Chen L. The evidence for opioid-induced hyperalgesia today. Austin J Anesth Analg. 2014;2:1024.
4. Schnell SA, Christie MJ, Vaughan CW, Marinelli S, Wessendorf MW. Rostral ventromedial medulla neurons that project to the spinal cord express multiple opioid receptor phenotypes. J Neurosci. 2002;22:10847–55.
5. Noueihed R, Yaksh TL. The physiology and pharmacology of spinal opiates. Annu Rev Pharmacol Toxicol. 1985;25:433–62.
6. Birnbaumer L, Abramowitz J, Brown AM. Receptor-effector coupling by G proteins. Biochim Biophys Acta. 1990;1031:163.
7. Roeske WR, Yamamura HI, Rubenzik MK, Sugiyama M, Rice KC, Varga EV, Stropova D, Grife V, Hruby VJ. Converging protein kinase pathways mediate adenylyl cyclase superactivation upon chronic delta-opioid agonist treatment. J Pharmacol Exp Ther. 2003;306:109–15.
8. Avidor-Reiss T, Nevo I, Levy R, Pfeuffer T, Vogel Z. Chronic opioid treatment induces adenylyl cyclase V superactivation. Involvement of Gbetagamma. J Biol Chem. 1996;271:21309.

Part II

Admission and Consultation

History

6

Rakhi Dayal

Key Points
- Dedicate enough time for detailed evaluation and review all available documents.
- Obtain a detailed history of the pain condition.
- Screen for red flags and yellow flags.
- Obtain a behavioral and psychological history.
- Select the appropriate pain rating tool for the patient.

History of Presenting Illness

When evaluating a patient's pain, review the patient's documents in detail to understand the underlying condition and the indication for the admission. Allocate sufficient time for interview and evaluation of the patient. Initiate the discussion with chief complaints and then obtain a detailed history of the presenting illness. Guide the patient to describe the pain onset, duration, location, radiation, nature and quality. Exacerbating and alleviating factors should be noted. Inquire about associated factors such as new onset neurological deficits such as weakness, urinary or bowel incontinence.

Pain Assessment Tools

There are several pain assessment tools available. Commonly used tools for adults are numeric rating scale, visual analogue scale and Wong Baker's scale. The FLACC [Face, Legs, Activity, Cry, Consolability] scale is useful for children under the age

R. Dayal (✉)
Department of Anesthesiology, University of California, Irvine, Orange, CA, USA
e-mail: rdayal@hs.uci.edu

© Springer Nature Switzerland AG 2022
D. A. Edwards et al. (eds.), *Hospitalized Chronic Pain Patient*,
https://doi.org/10.1007/978-3-031-08376-1_6

of 8 years. For patients with barriers to communication such as an infant, intubated patient, or a patient with dementia separate scales are available, which should be referred to.

Establish the patient's baseline pain, if any and differentiate how the current pain is different in severity or presentation. In chronic pain patients, this is helpful to establish reasonable goals of treatment.

Functional Status

Obtain details of the functional status before and after the presenting pain; the goal being to restore or improve functionality.

Past Medical History/Past Surgical History

Past medical history and past surgical history should be reviewed to get an overview of the patient's comorbid conditions. Severity of the comorbidities may need to be evaluated as certain comorbidities may place the individual at higher risk of complication with therapeutic pain modalities. In which case, they should be avoided, and alternatives considered.

Medication List

Obtain and review the patient's current medication list for appropriateness and interactions. Confirm the dosage and frequency of the medication. It is useful to ask if the patient notices any side effects of the medications. Obtain a history of the pain medications tried in the past including the ones that failed. This will help in generating the treatment plan. Of note, most chronic pain patients have a physician responsible for the recurrent assessment and treatment management. Contact details of the physician are helpful in coordinating care. For controlled substances, the medications should be verified with the state prescription drug-monitoring program. If the patient is from another state, efforts should be made to contact the last treating physician for medication reconciliation. This is also a good time to review the anticoagulant medications, which need to be kept in mind for planning any therapeutic intervention as a nerve or neuraxial block.

Review of Systems

Since the admission is usually for a medical or surgical reason, review any recent clinical or medication changes, which may exacerbate the patient's comorbidities or cause other organ dysfunction.

Psychological History

Many chronic pain patients have concurrent depression or another psychological condition. If the psychological presentation is considered an impediment to the improvement in the patient's pain condition appropriate resources should be offered. History of suicidal ideation should be evaluated further by defining if the condition is active or remote. Family history of psychological disorders, suicide or substance misuse is important and may have an association with the patient's psychological health. History of substance or alcohol misuse should be well documented. Inquire if it is recent or remote. Support the patient's rehabilitation with due consideration when considering medications that have an addiction potential.

Special Considerations

Implantable Pain Devices: Spinal Cord Stimulator and Intrathecal Drug Delivery Device

If a patient has an implanted device for pain—inquire if it is a stimulator or intrathecal drug delivery device. The patients usually have an information card that would be helpful in identifying the device and the manufacturing company. It would also have a phone number to contact for questions and support needed in management of the device. If the patient has an intrathecal device, inquire if the patient is aware of what medication is present in the pump, when they had the last refill, if there were any recent medication dosage changes and when the next refill is due. The device may have to be interrogated at that evaluation or efforts made to contact the patients pain provider for the most recent interrogation. If not, then consider an interrogation at the time of evaluation.

Post-Surgical Patients

Postsurgical patients recover at different pace depending on type of surgery and the patients' clinical condition. Common milestones to inquire about is if patient has regained his bowel function. History of passing flatus or stools is reassuring. Oral medications can be initiated if the patient is tolerating their diet. Inquire if the patient can ambulate and/or participate in physical therapy. This is an important part of recovery and deep vein thrombosis prevention. Inquire if the limitations are associated with pain.

Patients with an Epidural

In a patient with an epidural, it is imperative to inquire about efficacy, coverage and possible adverse effects. Remote but possible complications are nerve injury, epidural hematoma and epidural abscess. Inquire about back pain, unanticipated weakness, systemic signs of infection. The epidural infusions usually consist of a combination of local anesthetic and opioid medication. Pharmacological adverse effects of neuraxial opioids may manifest as itching, constipation, sedation and shortness of breath. Local anesthetic adverse effects could be dizziness, numbness, weakness and palpitations to name a few.

Patients with a Peripheral Nerve Block

Assess for efficacy and adequacy of coverage of the targeted area. The patient may have received a one-time block or a continuous infusion catheter. Common issues may be soreness at the site or leaking around the catheter. Depending on the time and type of nerve block the patient may have motor weakness. Review the records to know the type of block and the time of the block to put the patient's symptoms in perspective. If the block was intended only for analgesia, motor weakness is unusual and warrants further investigation.

Summary

In as much as pain is a warning sign which alerts the patient and the physician to an underlying pathology, it is also an impediment to patient comfort, recovery and functionality. Advocating improved patient evaluation, assessment and therapeutic treatment plan can enable us to achieve our common goals of improve pain control.

Physical Examination

7

Rakhi Dayal

Key Points
- Detailed physical examination for thorough assessment of pain is essential.
- Neurological evaluation provides information that is useful for evaluation of patient and titration of therapeutic regimen.
- Epidural infusion and peripheral nerve blocks are unique modalities of analgesia that require special vigilance.
- Postsurgical evaluations need unique evaluation and attention to perioperative recovery.
- Adequate evaluation for pain should include the risk of misuse of medications.
- Re-evaluation of the patient's pain after an intervention or therapeutic change is instrumental in developing treatment recommendations for discharge.

Goals of the Exam

In general, the goals of physical examination for inpatient pain management of hospitalized patients are as follows:

- Determine the basis and evaluate the source of the pain.
- Provide useful data regarding the severity of presenting and comorbid conditions to assess the safety of initiating pharmacological or interventional pain modalities.
- Identify the effectiveness of ongoing pain interventions such as epidural infusion and peripheral nerve blockade.

R. Dayal (✉)
Department of Anesthesiology, University of California, Irvine, Orange, CA, USA
e-mail: rdayal@hs.uci.edu

© Springer Nature Switzerland AG 2022
D. A. Edwards et al. (eds.), *Hospitalized Chronic Pain Patient*,
https://doi.org/10.1007/978-3-031-08376-1_7

- Obtain a thorough neurological examination which is helpful in assessing for adverse effects associated with pain regimens, thereby guide further therapeutic decision making.
- Obtain a psychological evaluation of the patient to assess their attitude towards pain and establish a baseline.

The examination should start with the vital signs and proceed from head to toe. The pertinent relevance of the examination is detailed in each section below.

Vital Signs

All five vital signs can provide significant information. Review of medical information or patient report is helpful in establishing the patient's baseline. Any deviation from normal or baseline should be evaluated for ongoing pathologies, medication interactions or a change in the clinical condition. A concise summary of pain related impacts on vital signs are detailed below:

- Temperature: If elevated could be concerning for infection or inflammation. Usually, fever noted on the first postoperative day is an inflammatory response and not highly concerning for infection as long as all other parameters such as site inspection, white blood cell count and neutrophilic shift are within normal limits. After postoperative day 4 the concern for infection gets higher. The source of infection may be localized such as urinary tract infection related to Foley catheter placement or more systemic. The possibility of infection is important to bear in mind to understand the clinical progression of the patient and in decision making for continuing pain modalities such as epidural infusions for analgesia.
- Pulse rate: Tachycardia may be sign that the patient is experiencing pain. Bradycardia is a potential side effect of opioid medications. However, other differential diagnosis should be considered and evaluated.
- Blood pressure: May be elevated with pain or a side effect of medications such as serotonin norepinephrine reuptake inhibitors [SNRI's] and tricyclic antidepressants. Low blood pressure may be secondary to the sympathetic blockade caused by epidural anesthesia, as local anesthetics are often used in the infusion.
- Respiratory rate decrease, increase and poor saturation may all be concerning. They all signify respiratory distress which should be closely considered when formulating the patient's treatment plan. For acute pain, the doses of opioid medications used are significantly higher than in chronic pain management. Sometimes the doses are escalated rapidly for therapeutic effect and pharmacologically the patients do not have the opportunity to develop tolerance. The consequence may be respiratory depression.
- Pain Score is a helpful tool in evaluating the patient's pain. It ranges from 0 to 10. Zero referring to "no pain" and 10/10 referring to the "worst pain". 1–3/10 implies mild pain, 4–6/10 moderate and 7–10/10 severe pain. The patient should be asked to rate the pain at baseline, when resting and with movement.

- Body mass index (BMI): High BMI can be associated with snoring or obstructive sleep apnea. These potentially increase the risk of inadequate oxygenation and possibly respiratory depression with opioids and other sedative medications.

Head and Neck Evaluation

- Eyes: Miosis may be seen when the patient is receiving opioid medications.
- Neck mass: Presence of large goiter, radiation changes or thick neck put the patient at potential risk of respiratory distress which may be compounded by pain pharmacological interventions.
- Airway assessment: General airway assessment is helpful. If the patient has a difficult airway or a cause for respiratory dysfunction, extreme caution should be used in using medications that may have a sedative or respiratory depression effect.

Neurological Examination

- Level of consciousness: Is the patient alert, awake and responsive? If not, this should be compared with what is documented in the chart and what is reported by the patient's family and friends as the patient's baseline. If there is an acute change, urgent/emergent medical attention and review of medications administered may be warranted.
- Orientation and memory changes: It is not unusual to see patients developing delirium or altered mental status when admitted in the hospital. Also, it is not unusual that patients with poor cognition and altered mental status present with conditions which inflict pain. Evaluate thoroughly to get a good assessment of the baseline.
- Sensory and motor testing: Commonly done for patients with spine pain, nerve related injury or pain and neurological changes. For patient with epidural or peripheral nerve block for analgesia it is not unusual to find decreased sensation in the dermatomes that are blocked. However, motor weakness is unlikely unless the block was intended for surgical anesthesia. New onset motor weakness is a pathognomonic sign, hence requires urgent evaluation and workup.
- Mood: Depression, anxiety and anger can all present with pain.
- Behavior Assessment: Patients who view pain as a weakness may be more likely to suffer with pain and present with other somatic complaints [1].

Skin Examination

- Patients with pain may present with changes is in sensitivity to a noxious or non-noxious stimulus.
- Assess for hyperalgesia, allodynia, hyperesthesia, and dysesthesia.

- Erythema and skin discoloration may be noted at the site of pain.
- Hair of growth changes may be noted in relation to underlying chronic pain condition (e.g., complex regional pain syndrome).
- Itching is more commonly noted with neuraxial opioids than systemic opioids.

Cardiovascular Examination

- Inspection: skin color for adequacy of perfusion
- Palpation: rate, rhythm of pulse
- Auscultation for carotid bruit and cardiac murmurs as deemed appropriate

Respiratory Examination

- Inspection for chest wall movement, general comfort of breathing or any notable distress.
- Positions such as an upright position is maintained by patients experiencing respiratory distress.
- They may also have difficulty in speaking in complete sentences.
- Percussion for consolidation or air-filled cavity.
- Palpation for subcutaneous crepitus as it can be present in trauma patients.
- Auscultation for wheeze or added sounds.

Abdominal Examination

- In addition to abdominal pathologies that present with pain, patients tend to develop ileus postoperatively or with the use of opioid medications.
- Inspection: distention, deformities, mass and surgical incision.
- Palpation: consistency, tenderness and rebound tenderness.
- Percussion: tympanic sound.
- Auscultation for bowel sounds.

Genitourinary Examination

- Sudden drop in the urinary output may suggest onset of renal dysfunction, thereby necessitating renal dosing for the medications.
- There is evidence that thoracic epidurals are unlikely to cause urinary retention, but lumbar epidurals may do so, hence necessitating Foley placement.
- Urinary retention may also occur from opioids and tricyclic antidepressants.

Extremity Examination

- Inspection for swelling, color changes, mass or deformity.
- Palpate for tenderness, capillary refill.
- Sensory and motor examination as deemed necessary.
- For patients with a splint, neurovascular assessment should be done.

Musculoskeletal Examination

- Spine: Inspection of the spine for general posture, alignment, symmetry, deformities, scars, muscle hypertrophy or atrophy. Evaluate the spine in flexion, extension and rotation to assess the range of motion. Palpation of the spinous processes may elicit tenderness or a step off. A step off may be suggestive of spondylolisthesis. A localized tenderness may be elicited over a spine fracture. Palpation of the muscles in the area may reproduce tenderness suggesting myofascial etiology of the pain.
  - Provocation tests include:
       Spurling's test (for cervical radiculopathy),
       straight leg raise test (for lumbar radiculopathy),
       FABER test (for sacroiliac joint dysfunction),
       FAIR's test (for piriformis syndrome), and
       KEMP test (for lumbar spondylosis).
  - Red flag signs would indicate emergent evaluation and consideration for intervention. These signs are saddle anesthesia, loss of anal sphincter tone, major motor weakness in lower extremities, fever, vertebral tenderness, limited range of motion and neurological findings persisting beyond 1 month [2]
- Joint Examination:
  - Inspection: swelling, erythema, masses and deformity
  - Palpation: warmth [concern for infection, fluctuant (suggestive of effusion)
  - Range of motion of the proximal and distal joint in addition to the joint under consideration
  - Specific tests: to assess for impingement, dislocation, meniscus or ligament injury should be conducted

Examination of Surgical Site

- Inspection for the extent of the incision—to get an idea of the site involved and to assess for adequate coverage with a regional anesthesia procedure.
- Assessing whether healing is progressing as expected is helpful in making adjustments in the pain treatment plan and to decide how long the epidural or peripheral nerve catheter may be needed.

- Collaboration with the primary team in the decision making is imperative.
- Erythema, discharge, wound vacuum or drains at the site could be concerning for infection and possibly worsening pain.
- Palpation around the site may be helpful in assessing for effusion or cellulitis. Tenderness may be elicited. Of note chest tubes tend to cause significant pain.

Examinations of Epidural Analgesia

- Site of epidural: check for erythema around the tape and under it. Ensure that the dressing is not soaked or coming off. If so, reinforcement of dressing or completely redoing the dressing may be required. The epidural insertion site should not be indurated or erythematous. Induration is suggestive of possible migration of the catheter, thereby leading to accumulation of the infusion under that site. Erythema may be a reaction to tape, pressure from catheter or infection. Discharge could be reflective of superficial or deep infection.
- Connection and integrity of the epidural catheter should be intact. The epidural catheter should have a yellow label indicating that it is an epidural. The epidural infusion tubing is uniquely colored yellow. There should be a filter between the epidural catheter and the infusion cassette.
- Infusion Medication: Check the epidural infusion pump medication and the settings. If the patient is using patient controlled analgesia, the infusion logs can be reviewed to get details of the frequency of medication utilization by the patient.
- Palpation of the back may or may not elicit pain. Mild to moderate pain may be present if the placement was difficult. Excruciating pain may be a sign of epidural hematoma.
- Assess the targeted area for concurrent coverage by testing with cold or pin prick technique. In general, there is a two-dermatome level difference between the sympathetic, sensory and motor levels, in that order.
- Indicators of complications such as epidural hematoma, abscess or nerve injury can be picked up on a complete neurological evaluation. Any change from the patient baseline warrants detailed evaluation.

Examination of Peripheral Nerve Blocks

- If it was a single shot nerve block the patient may or may not have sensory or motor residual effect depending on the time at which the injection was done. Depending on the pharmacological duration of the medication the blocks may last and hour to 12 h.
- If the patient has a continuous infusion catheter, there could be various types of pumps that are used for the infusion. Appropriate settings and medication concentration should be verified.

- The type of block would dictate the necessary components of the examination. In general, infection, hematoma or peri-catheter site leak are common complications of nerve blocks.
- Potential but relatively rare complications are local anesthetic toxicity, nerve injury, vascular injury or block failure [3].

In addition to the above, there unique nuances of each block which the provider should be aware of. Some of these are detailed below:

- Interscalene block: pneumothorax, block or injury of surrounding nerves (e.g., phrenic nerve, recurrent laryngeal nerve and vagal nerve). There may be occasion spread of the local anesthetic in the neuraxial space causing concerns of epidural or intrathecal spread of the local anesthetic. There is also a possibility of injury to the vessels such as carotid or vertebral artery or the internal/external jugular vein.
- Supraclavicular brachial plexus block: pneumothorax, brachial plexus injury, injury to subclavian vein or artery.
- Infraclavicular: pneumothorax, brachial plexus injury, vascular injury.
- Axillary nerve block: nerve or vascular injury.
- Intercostal nerve block: High chance of local anesthetic toxicity especially if several levels are done.
- Transversus abdominal plane block: visceral injury.
- Lumbar plexus block: neuraxial spread of local anesthetic. Concern for vascular injury and hematoma is higher than other peripheral nerve blocks.
- Femoral nerve block: quadriceps weakness which may interfere with rehabilitation and increase the risk of fall.
- Adductor canal block: a modification of the femoral nerve block which prevents the likelihood of quadriceps weakness and thereby the risk of fall.
- Sciatic nerve block: This can be done high up in the thigh or at the level of the popliteal fossa.

Summary

A detailed physical examination is important for initial evaluation of the patient to correlate the patients presenting symptoms with appropriate signs to establish an appropriate diagnosis. Patients should be re-evaluated at appropriate intervals to assess the improvement or side effects with the recommended interventions. Focused physical examination should be done at time of re-evaluation. In general, sedation precedes respiratory depression with opioid medications. If the patient is sedated in still reporting 10/10 pain on the numeric rating scale, expert clinical judgment should be used in developing the treatment plan.

References

1. Li JM. Pain management in the hospitalized patient. Med Clin N Am. 2008;92(2):371–85.
2. Bratton RL. Assessment and management of acute low back pain. Am Fam Physician. 1999;60(8):2299–308.
3. Jeng CL, Torrillo TM, Rosenblatt MA. Complications of peripheral nerve blocks. Br J Anaesth. 2010;105(Suppl 1):i97–107.

The SCRIPT History Template

Stephanie G. Vanterpool

8

Introduction

Gathering a concise, yet accurate and complete pain history from a patient can be very challenging. This is often due to a combination of both patient-related and provider-related factors. Patient-related factors include being a poor historian or providing incomplete information. Provider-related factors may include not knowing what to ask, or not knowing how to resolve things that do not make sense. Often, the history we are able to obtain comes out in a jumbled fashion, similar to a bowl of puzzle pieces. So how can we turn those puzzle pieces of a patient's history into a recognizable picture?

The answer may lie in the use of a pain specific history template—the S.C.R.I.P.T. history. The benefits of using a history template are already well established in other disease and patient settings, such as emergency medicine [1]. A template allows for a logical progression of data and allows the clinician to plug in information as it is obtained, while ensuring that key components are not missed. The S.C.R.I.P.T history template consists of five main sections (Table 8.1):

Story: This is where the circumstances of onset of pain are elicited. In a hospitalized patient this may include recent surgery (post-op patient), trauma (fall, motor vehicle accident, etc.), or other systemic illness. It is also important to document the baseline pain state for the patient—is there a history of chronic pain, or recurring acute pain exacerbations? What is the location of the patient's typical pain, and what is the typical severity, treatment regimen, etc.?

Current symptoms: The current symptoms are the typical components of a history—Location, description, severity, aggravating, and alleviating factors. In a

S. G. Vanterpool (✉)
Department of Anesthesiology, University of Tennessee Graduate School of Medicine, Knoxville, TN, USA
e-mail: svanterpool@utmck.edu

© Springer Nature Switzerland AG 2022
D. A. Edwards et al. (eds.), *Hospitalized Chronic Pain Patient*,
https://doi.org/10.1007/978-3-031-08376-1_8

Table 8.1 The S.C.R.I.P.T. history template—hospitalized patient

S.C.R.I.P.T	Information to gather	What it highlights
Story	– Circumstances of onset (acute, trauma, surgery, insidious, etc.) – Chronic baseline pain? Same or different? – Mental status? – Details, Details, Details	– Mechanism of injury – Psychosocial component
Current symptoms	– Pain location (precise anatomic location) – Pain description (burning, tingling, aching, throbbing, etc.) – Aggravating factors Alleviating factors	– Pain states – Anatomic causes
Rx (Relevant Meds)	– Anti-inflammatories, muscle relaxants, nerve pain medication – Home medication regimen (continued in hospital?)	– Pain mechanisms
Intervention	– Previous injections to the area (what was injected, what type of injection was done?) – Recent surgery? Complications? Other?	– Anatomic causes
Physical therapy	– Previous physical activity level – Activity while hospitalized (inpatient PT? Out of bed? Ambulation?)	– Functional causes
Tests	– Imaging of the affected area, Doppler studies, NCS/EMG, etc. (if done), lab work?	– Anatomic causes – Physiologic causes

hospitalized patient it is important to clarify location in particular as the cause of the acute pain may be different from any known chronic or post-operative pain.

Rx (Relevant Medications): Be sure to document any home medications for pain, and whether the patient is still receiving them or an equivalent in the hospital. Also document the current acute pain medication regimen, and what is actually being administered to the patient, not just what is ordered. Include non-opioid medications (both home and inpatient) such as muscle relaxers, neuromodulators, anti-inflammatory medications. And note any other relevant medications being administered in the hospital such as anticoagulants, GI prophylaxis, systemic steroids, etc.

Interventions: For the hospitalized patient, interventions may include recent surgeries, injections or other procedures performed as an outpatient or during this hospitalization. These may include interventions both to address the pain complaint (e.g., Diagnostic laparoscopy for abdominal pain), or that may have preceded the pain compliant/presentation.

Physical therapy/activity: Has the patient been physically active immediately preceding the onset of pain? Is there deconditioning, immobility, or some other form of functional decline contributing to the pain complaint? Has the patient been ordered inpatient PT? Have they participated in physical activity or therapy (out of bed, walking, etc.)?

Tests: What imaging or diagnostic testing is available and already on the chart? Is the imaging or diagnostic testing that is available consistent with the suspected cause of pain? If not, what else may help elicit the underlying cause of pain?

Pain Red Flags

Pain red flags are findings on patient assessment that should trigger you to look for a more accurate cause of the pain. These red flags are broadly applicable to all types of pain, not just spine or low back pain [2]. Often these red flags can be grouped into three broad categories:

1. Pain outside of the expected location. Should prompt more detailed physical examination
   (a) E.g., A patient who is post-op day 2 from a bowel resection, now complaining of pain in the left leg.
2. Pain out of proportion to the working diagnosis: Prompts the evaluator to ask the question - does this working diagnosis still apply to the observed situation?
   (a) E.g., A patient with recurrent cellulitis due to a history of IV drug use, but now in visible acute distress and complaining of 10/10 pain with unstable vital signs.
3. "Something's not right" - A catch all red flag that prompts the evaluator to connect the available information and ensure that a logical sequence of events or proposed pathophysiology can be identified
   (a) E.g., a patient with right leg weakness causing frequent falls, but MRI from 1 year ago shows only mild L4/5 disc bulge.

It is beneficial to have a systematic process to resolve these red flags when present. This process includes five steps:

Step 1. Re-visit the story—make sure you are not missing anything

Step 2. Clarify the current symptoms—location, radiation, sensation, etc.

Step 3. Repeat the physical exam

Step 4. Evaluate existing tests

Step 5. Order new tests if needed.

Remember, presence of a Pain Red Flag should always prompt you to identify the *accurate diagnosis* and treat the *CAUSE* of the pain [3].

References

1. Marx J. Rosen's emergency medicine: concepts and clinical practice. 7th edition. Philadelphia: Mosby/Elsevier. 2010:pp. 267. ISBN 978-0-323-05472-0.
2. Samanta J, Kendall J, Samanta A. Chronic low back pain. BMJ. 2003;326:535. https://doi.org/10.1136/bmj.326.7388.535.
3. Vardeh D, Mannion RJ, Woolf CJ. Toward a mechanism-based approach to pain diagnosis. J Pain. 2016;17(9 Suppl):T50–69.

Patient Reported Outcomes

9

Michael Kent

Key Points
- Patient reported outcomes promote shared decision making, problem identification, and improved provider–patient communication.
- Multidimensional measures allow for a comprehensive characterization of patient's pain experience.
- Daily measures should include questions related to physical function, pain interference, and sleep at a minimum.
- NIH's PROMIS measures represent a comprehensive biopsychosocial health measurement system that has displayed equivalent if not better validity than many legacy measures.

Patient Reported Outcomes

Patient reported outcomes refer to the report of a patient's health condition (e.g., symptoms, function, etc.) or experience that comes directly from the patient (or surrogate) without interpretation by a clinician [1, 2]. The use of PROs has been well documented in outcomes research (e.g., comparative effectiveness, etc.) with an evolving ability to provide individualized care and, in aggregate, to yield measures of performance [3, 4]. A vast array of pain related PROs currently exists highlighting the concept that PROs cannot be isolated from the resources needed to implement them.

In general, beyond required validity and reliability, successful PROs share the key characteristics of being simple, brief, sensitive to change, informed by patients, and easily interpreted. Additionally, a thorough implementation strategy is key for workflow integration and systems-based integration (Table 9.1).

M. Kent (✉)
Department of Anesthesiology, Duke University Health System, Durham, NC, USA

© Springer Nature Switzerland AG 2022
D. A. Edwards et al. (eds.), *Hospitalized Chronic Pain Patient*,
https://doi.org/10.1007/978-3-031-08376-1_9

Table 9.1 Institutional considerations for PRO implementation

Key Institutional Questions for PRO Implementation
What are your goals for collecting PROs in your clinical practice and what resources are available?
Which groups of patients will you assess?
How do you select which questionnaire to use?
How often should patients complete questionnaires?
How will the PROs be administered and scored?
When/Where/How will results be presented?
Who will receive score reports?
What will be done to respond to issues identified through the PROs?
How will the value of using PROs be evaluated?

Adapted content from International Society for Quality of Life Research report titled User's Guide to Implementing Patient-Reported Outcomes Assessment in Clinical Practice [5]

PROs in the Hospitalized Chronic Pain Patient

General Strategy

Utilizing PROs for the surveillance, measurement, and tracking of pain in a hospitalized chronic pain patient with or without acute pain must focus on multidimensional variables (e.g., pain interference, physical function, pain behavior, pain intensity, etc.). Unidimensional pain intensity ratings (e.g., Numerical Rating Scale, Visual Analog Scale, etc.) alone are of limited value. Ideally, baseline measurements are available prior to admission. A key decision point pertains to the choice of PROs that focus on acute pain and those that focus on the patient's chronic pain condition. A systems-based focus where chosen PROs can be utilized in both an inpatient and outpatient setting is key in providing comprehensive and effective transitional pain care. Minimization of response burden is also a key consideration in this setting as well.

Frequency of Administration

A variety of PROs are available in the acute and chronic pain setting. PROs in the acute setting are often administered on a 24-h basis whereas PROs in the chronic setting are administered at a variety of times points (weeks, months). Further, pain-centric PROs are often psychometrically validated over a given timeframe such as "over the last 24 h" or "over the last 7 days.". Choice of PRO must take into account such limits and timeframe.

Specific Choice of Instrument

Domain Selection

A variety of biopsychosocial measures modulate acute and chronic pain experiences. Measures such as physical function, pain interference, depression, anxiety, or pain catastrophizing have clear links to the pain experience. However, consideration of other biopsychosocial measures such as self-efficacy, anger, and social satisfaction should be considered as applicable to the hospitalized chronic pain patient. Prior to administration, teams must not only choose which domains are _applicable_ to their patient population but which domains they wish to measure on a _daily_ interval versus domains they wish to administer at _remote_ intervals.

Daily Instruments (Table 9.2)

- Unidimensional: Pain intensity scales such as the Visual Analog Scale (0–100 mm), the Numerical Rating Scale (0–10), or the Verbal Description Scale (No Pain, Mild, Moderate, Severe, and Excruciating) are available valid and reliable measures [6]. In clinical practice, the Numerical Rating Scale (NRS), is the most commonly utilized scale within the inpatient setting. The NRS has a long history of established reliability and validity. Specifically, the NRS has acceptable discriminative capability but also enough options to have the ability to detect change over time. However, while the NRS is an important tool, its unidimensional nature significantly limits the characterization of the multidimensional nature of pain.
- Multidimensional:

  Defense and Veterans Pain Rating Scale (DVPRS): Stemming from the limitations of unidimensional pain intensity scales, the Defense and Veterans Pain Rating Scale was developed in a joint Department of Defense and Veteran's Health Administration effort. The DVPRS expands on the NRS by integrating visual variables (faces/colors) along with descriptive functional anchors assigned to pain intensity designations. Additionally, four additional supplemental questions focused on sleep, anxiety, activity, and mood offer further information regarding the impact of pain. Such a tool is quickly administered at the bedside and can be administered on a daily basis. While new within the landscape of pain related patient reported outcomes, the DVPRS scale was found to have acceptable reliability and validity in a sample of 350 inpatient/outpatient active duty or retired military personnel [7].

  Brief Pain Inventory Short Form (BPI- SF): The Brief Pain Inventory—Short Form is a reliable and validated tool consisting of 9 items focused on pain severity and its inherent impact on daily functioning [8]. Numerous interference items

Table 9.2 Daily instruments

Daily measurements		
Instrument	Scale	Comments
Unidimensional		
NRS	1–10	– Most widely applied pain intensity measure
VRS	No pain, mild, moderate, severe, excruciating	– Less discriminative capability
VAS	0–100 mm	– Difficult bedside administration
Multidimensional		
DVPRS	5 item	– Used for surgical/non-surgical populations
		– Easy bedside administration
		– Measures include Pain Intensity/Interference, Sleep, Activity, Mood, Stress
		– No scoring required
		– Administration time: <2 min–
		– May be administered on 24 h basis
BPI-SF	15 item	– Administration time: 5 min
		– Measures include pain intensity, pain relief, general activity, mood, sleep, walking, work, social relations, enjoyment of life
		– Subscale scoring available
QoR- 15 or 40	15 or 40 items	– Intended for post-surgical recovery
		– Scoring utilized or individual item examination possible
		– Administration time: 2 min
		– May be administered on 24 h basis
SF-36	36 Items	– Does not address sleep
		– Mostly used in research or large comparison setting
		– Scoring required and subscale scoring available
		– Administration time: 10 min

include sleep, general activity, mood, walking, work, personal relations, and enjoyment of life. The BPI SF is a shorter version of the long form BPI which contains further clinical adjectives but increases response burden.

Quality of Recovery (9, 15 or 40 items): Specific to recovery after surgery, multidimensional recovery scales are available and applicable to a post-surgical population with chronic pain. Both scales cover approximately 5–6 multidimensional domains such as physical comfort, physical independence, emotional state, etc. and are indexed over 24 h [9, 10]. While administration and examination of individual items can be useful, scoring is utilized with minimal important changes of 0.9, 8, and 6.3 for the QoR-9 scores, QoR 15, and QoR 40 respectively [11].

Longitudinal Instruments

A variety of pain related patient reported outcomes are not ideal for daily administration either due to unlikely daily change (e.g., depression, pain catastrophizing, etc.) or construction of the measure (e.g., "…over the last 7 days", ".… Since admission"). However, baseline and follow up measurement of such outcomes provides a valuable interaction to establish a longitudinal relationship with the hospitalized chronic pain patient to ensure a structured transition to the outpatient arena where such PROs can be continued.

NIH's Patient Reported Outcomes Measurement Information System (PROMIS—www.healthmeasures.net)

Due to the lack of standardized health measures, the NIH has invested over US$100 million spanning over a decade of effort in order to develop a comprehensive system of health-related PRO item banks. Leveraging item response theory and computer adaptive testing, PROMIS item banks offer significant precision with minimal response burden. PROMIS measures have shown to have just as good if not better validity when compared to legacy scales [12]. PROMIS measures contain a variety of pain related item banks to include pain interference, physical function, or pain behavior and numerous item banks of measures that modulate the pain experience (e.g., anxiety, anger, depression, etc.). PROMIS measures represent a significant advancement in the precision and standardization of health measures. All PROMIS measures are scored via a "t score" with a mean of 50 and a standard deviation of 10 and underwent calibration via large samples of the US general population. A higher t score translates to a patient having more of a certain measure. For example, a patient may have a high depression t score correlating to poorer health unlike a patient that may have a higher physical function t score correlating to better health. Most measures are indexed "…over the last 7 days" and this should be taken into consideration when applied to the inpatient setting. However, PROMIS measures allow providers to longitudinally "speak the same language" which provides significant value as such measures can be instituted in the inpatient setting and continued into the outpatient phase of care. Of significant importance, PROMIS measures can be administered via computer adaptive testing or by short form.

Legacy Measures: While PROMIS measures represent an immense leap forward in the capability to capture measures of health and pain, a variety of well validated multidimensional pain related measures are also available. Of note, other than Pain Catastrophizing, PROMIS measures have shown to be equivalent in validity when compared to the below legacy measures. While many biopsychosocial modulators are known, the below list represents a list of commonly measured items.

- Pain Catastrophizing: Pain catastrophizing has been linked to numerous outcomes including increased acute/chronic pain scores, increase opioid use, and delayed pain resolution [13–15]. Currently the pain catastrophizing scales (PCS) can be administered at any time point (prehospitalization vs. post hospitalization) but its utility at follow up time points has not been established.
- Depression and Anxiety: Depression and anxiety maintain a strong link to both acute and chronic pain and are essential measurements in any hospitalized patient in pain [16, 17]. While baseline measurement prior to hospitalization is ideal,

measurement in the inpatient setting can enhance immediate pain care and establish longitudinal surveillance. Example scales that include depression are the Patient Health Questionnaire 9 item or the Center for Epidemiologic Studies Depression Scale. Scales that include anxiety are Generalized Anxiety Disorder 7 item or the Hospital Anxiety and Depression Scale
- Sleep Interference: Sleep interference/disturbance plays an essential role in pain modulation in both the acute and chronic setting [18]. A variety of measures are available for daily and remote surveillance.
- Pain Resilience: While recognizing as a modulating measure in chronic pain, pain resilience has also emerged as a possible mediator in acute pain states. A recent scale showing good construct and predictive validity is the Pain Resilience Scale [19].

Conclusion

Patient reported outcomes serve as a foundation in the care of the acute or chronic pain patient. While objective and biologic markers of the pain experience are essential, patient reported outcome allow providers to tailor analgesic regimens to patient's biopsychosocial experience allowing for the creation of longitudinal relationships. Further, patient reported outcomes allow for a focus on the biopsychosocial impact of the pain experience to assist in patient stratification and intervention in not only pain etiology but mediators as well.

References

1. Bream E, Charman SC, Clift B, Murray D, Black N. Relationship between patients' and clinicians' assessments of health status before and after knee arthroplasty. Qual Saf Health Care. 2010;19(6):e6. https://doi.org/10.1136/qshc.2008.031310. Epub 2010 Jul 1. PMID: 20595715.
2. Deshpande PR, Rajan S, Sudeepthi BL, Abdul Nazir CP. Patient-reported outcomes: a new era in clinical research. Perspect Clin Res. 2011;2(4):137–44.
3. Tunis SR, Clarke M, Gorst SL, et al. Improving the relevance and consistency of outcomes in comparative effectiveness research. J Comp Eff Res. 2016;5(2):193–205.
4. Basch E, Spertus J, Dudley RA, et al. Methods for developing patient-reported outcome-based performance measures (PRO-PMs). Value Health. 2015;18(4):493–504.
5. Snyder CF, Aaronson NK, Choucair AK, et al. Implementing patient-reported outcomes assessment in clinical practice: a review of the options and considerations. Qual Life Res. 2012;21(8):1305–14.
6. Hjermstad MJ, Fayers PM, Haugen DF, et al. Studies comparing Numerical Rating Scales, Verbal Rating Scales, and Visual Analogue Scales for assessment of pain intensity in adults: a systematic literature review. J Pain Symptom Manag. 2011;41(6):1073–93.
7. Polomano RC, Galloway KT, Kent ML, et al. Psychometric Testing of the Defense and Veterans Pain Rating Scale (DVPRS): a new pain scale for military population. Pain Med. 2016;17(8):1505–19.
8. Mendoza T, Mayne T, Rublee D, Cleeland C. Reliability and validity of a modified Brief Pain Inventory short form in patients with osteoarthritis. Eur J Pain. 2006;10(4):353–61.

9. Gornall BF, Myles PS, Smith CL, et al. Measurement of quality of recovery using the QoR-40: a quantitative systematic review. Br J Anaesth. 2013;111(2):161–9.
10. Stark PA, Myles PS, Burke JA. Development and psychometric evaluation of a postoperative quality of recovery score: the QoR-15. Anesthesiology. 2013;118(6):1332–40.
11. Myles PS, Myles DB, Galagher W, Chew C, MacDonald N, Dennis A. Minimal clinically important difference for three quality of recovery scales. Anesthesiology. 2016;125(1):39–45.
12. Fries JF, Bruce B, Cella D. The promise of PROMIS: using item response theory to improve assessment of patient-reported outcomes. Clin Exp Rheumatol. 2005;23(5 Suppl 39):S53–7.
13. Schreiber KL, Kehlet H, Belfer I, Edwards RR. Predicting, preventing and managing persistent pain after breast cancer surgery: the importance of psychosocial factors. Pain Manag. 2014;4(6):445–59.
14. Sobol-Kwapinska M, Bąbel P, Plotek W, Stelcer B. Psychological correlates of acute postsurgical pain: a systematic review and meta-analysis. Eur J Pain. 2016;20(10):1573–86.
15. Harrison AM, McCracken LM, Bogosian A, Moss-Morris R. Towards a better understanding of MS pain: a systematic review of potentially modifiable psychosocial factors. J Psychosom Res. 2015;78(1):12–24.
16. Ghoneim MM, O'Hara MW. Depression and postoperative complications: an overview. BMC Surg. 2016;16(1):5.
17. Hooten WM. Chronic pain and mental health disorders: shared neural mechanisms, epidemiology, and treatment. Mayo Clin Proc. 2016;91(7):955–70.
18. Axén I. Pain-related sleep disturbance: a prospective study with repeated measures. Clin J Pain. 2016;32(3):254–9.
19. Slepian PM, Ankawi B, Himawan LK, France CR. Development and initial validation of the pain resilience scale. J Pain. 2016;17(4):462–72.

Clinical and Experimental Tools for Measuring Pain

10

Kristen M. Woods and Burel R. Goodin

Introduction

Chronic pain is a subjective, complex, and varied experience across patients. As such, clinicians and researchers have encountered substantial difficulties in measuring pain in a reliable and valid manner [1]. One of the now commonly incorporated methods for dealing with this pain measurement difficulty is the use of experimental pain stimuli to simulate patients' pain experience. The use of experimental pain stimuli for this purpose is collectively referred to as quantitative sensory testing (QST). The focus of this chapter is to provide an introduction to QST, including a focused discussion of methodology and evidence regarding the relationship of QST response measures to chronic pain. For detailed information, readers are referred to other, more comprehensive reviews of this topic [2–4]. It has been suggested that QST may be useful for the following:

- Characterize the anatomic and physiologic basis of normal and pathological sensory and pain perception [2, 3].
- Discern differences among chronic pain conditions that have clinically similar presentations [5].
- Generation of pain modulation profiles that can inform a patient's risk (or resilience) for poor chronic pain outcomes [6, 7].
- Evaluate patients' responses to pharmacologic and non-pharmacologic treatment [8, 9].

K. M. Woods
Department of Medicine, University of Alabama at Birmingham, Birmingham, AL, USA

B. R. Goodin (✉)
Department of Psychology, University of Alabama at Birmingham, Birmingham, AL, USA

Department of Anesthesiology and Perioperative Medicine, University of Alabama at Birmingham, Birmingham, AL, USA
e-mail: bgoodin1@uab.edu

© Springer Nature Switzerland AG 2022
D. A. Edwards et al. (eds.), *Hospitalized Chronic Pain Patient*,
https://doi.org/10.1007/978-3-031-08376-1_10

QST Methodology

Stimulus Modalities and Target Tissues

Multiple different stimulus modalities are generally included as part of an overall QST battery used to assess human pain perception. A multimodal approach is advantageous because these various modalities engage different nerve fibers, different components of afferent somatosensory transmission, and central nervous system pathways involved in processing painful stimuli [2]. Thermal (heat, cold) and mechanical (pressure) stimuli are perhaps the most frequently employed modalities; however, electrical, ischemic, and chemical stimulation are also used. Thermal heat stimulation can be accomplished by applying a contact probe to the skin surface, while thermal cold stimulation often involves submerging a part of the body into refrigerated water (i.e., immersion). Most QST procedures stimulate cutaneous tissue; however, other tissues can be targeted including myofascial and visceral organs (e.g., uterine cervix, esophagus). A recent review of QST methods provides additional detail regarding QST stimulus modalities and their characteristics [3]. Table 10.1 presents a list of typical stimulus modalities as well as the target tissues they stimulate.

Table 10.1 Types of QST stimulus modalities, the tissues they stimulate, and the response measures that are captured by each modality

Stimulus modality	Tissue stimulated	QST response measures
Thermal (contact heat)	Cutaneous	Pain threshold
		Pain tolerance
		Suprathreshold pain responses
		Temporal summation of pain
Thermal (immersion cold)	Cutaneous	Pain threshold
	Myofascial	Pain tolerance
		Suprathreshold pain responses
Mechanical (pressure)	Cutaneous	Pain threshold
	Myofascial	Pain tolerance
	Visceral	Suprathreshold pain responses
		Temporal summation of pain
Chemical (hypertonic saline, capsaicin)	Cutaneous	Allodynia[a]
	Myofascial	Hyperalgesia[b]
		Suprathreshold pain responses
Ischemic	Myofascial	Pain threshold
		Pain tolerance
		Suprathreshold pain responses
Electrical	Cutaneous	Pain threshold
	Myofascial	Pain tolerance
	Visceral	Suprathreshold pain responses
		Temporal summation of pain
Conditioned Pain Modulation	Cutaneous	Conditioned pain modulation is often measured with cold (immersion) as the conditioning stimulus and heat or pressure (contact) as the test stimulus
	Myofascial	

Adapted from (Cruz-Almeida 2014) [3]
[a]Allodynia refers to the experience of pain from a non-painful stimulus
[b]Hyperalgesia refers to exaggerated pain sensitivity

QST Response Measures

The QST response measures used to characterize human pain perception are frequently categorized as either "static" or "dynamic" in nature [10, 11]. Traditionally, QST has been used in a static way by measuring responses to single discrete stimuli with either fixed intensities or intensities that gradually change over time. More recently, advanced methods of dynamic QST have been developed whereby stimuli are applied repetitively or simultaneously to different body areas. Across an ever-increasing number of studies, dynamic QST response measures are emerging as more reliable and valid predictors of chronic pain outcomes than static measures [2]. However, the specific QST response measures assessed in a given setting should be tailored to the specific clinical or research question being asked.

Static and dynamic QST response measures are listed below. Table 10.1 also displays the QST response measures that can be obtained from each type of stimulus modalities.

Static

- Pain threshold refers to the intensity at which a stimulus is first perceived as painful.
- Pain tolerance refers to the maximum amount of pain produced by a stimulus that a person is able/willing to tolerate.
- Suprathreshold pain responses are ratings of pain in response to discrete stimuli with intensities above pain threshold detection. Numeric ratings scales are used to quantify the intensity of the suprathreshold pain. Patients provide an intensity rating using any number on 0–100 scale whereby 0 = no pain and 100 = the most intense pain imaginable.

Dynamic

- A routinely used QST protocol for the measurement of endogenous pain inhibition is conditioned pain modulation, which refers to the reduction in pain from one stimulus (the test stimulus) produced by the application of a second pain stimulus at a remote body site (the conditioning stimulus) [12]. Conditioned pain modulation is believed to reflect the perceptual manifestation of diffuse noxious inhibitory controls [13], whereby ascending projections from one noxious stimulus activate supraspinal structures that trigger descending inhibitory projections to the dorsal horn.
- Temporal summation of pain refers to a form of endogenous pain facilitation characterized by the perception of increased pain despite constant or even reduced peripheral afferent input [14]. Temporal summation is presumed to be the psychophysical manifestation of wind-up [15]. Wind-up is a phenomenon where repetitive stimulation of C primary afferents at rates greater than 0.3 Hz produces a slowly increasing response of second-order neurons in the spinal cord [16].

Clinical Relevance

Predicting Clinical Pain

QST response measures including (1) lower pain threshold, (2) lower pain tolerance, (3) exaggerated responses to suprathreshold painful stimuli, (4) greater temporal summation of pain, and (5) less efficient conditioned pain modulation consistently distinguish patients with chronic pain from healthy, pain-free controls [17]. Emerging evidence also suggests that QST response measures may also have value for prospectively predicting chronic pain development as well as the severity of chronic pain over time. For example, greater pre-surgical temporal summation of pain predicted the development of chronic pain 12 months following total knee arthroplasty in patients with knee osteoarthritis [18]. In patients who underwent thoracotomy, less efficient conditioned pain modulation measured pre-surgically predicted the development of chronic pain at the surgery site approximately 6 months following the procedure [19]. In studies that examined the associations of QST response measures with chronic pain severity, it was found that greater ratings of pain intensity in response to suprathreshold heat stimuli predicted more severe clinical pain in treatment-seeking patients with chronic shoulder pain [20]. Further, temporal summation of pain assessed at the hand and the knee significantly predicted weekly diary ratings of average clinical pain across 4 weeks in patients with knee osteoarthritis [21].

Predicting Treatment Responses

QST response measures have been found to predict pain treatment efficacy, and QST may also represent a useful marker of treatment outcome. In patients with postherpetic neuralgia, higher baseline heat pain thresholds predicted greater reduction in pain and higher ratings of pain relief in response to initiating a trial of controlled-release morphine sulfate [22]. In a study of painful diabetic neuropathy, results showed that patients with less efficient conditioned pain modulation (i.e., poor endogenous pain inhibition) prior to treatment initiation reported the greatest improvements in their pain severity in response to a trial of the duloxetine [23]. Further, treatment-induced improvement in conditioned pain modulation was correlated with duloxetine efficacy. In a separate study of diabetic peripheral neuropathy, patients received daily treatment with sustained-release tapentadol; conditioned pain modulation was measured before and after treatment [24]. Patients did not demonstrate significant conditioned pain modulation prior to treatment initiation; however, conditioned pain modulation was significantly activated by tapentadol at the end of the treatment trial. This activation of conditioned pain modulation coincided with significant pain alleviating effects of tapentadol. The authors concluded that the pain reducing effects of tapentadol in chronic pain patients with diabetic peripheral neuropathy was dependent on activation of endogenous pain inhibition as observed by conditioned pain modulation responses. It should be noted that the utility of QST measures for predicting treatment responses is not just limited to chronic neuropathic pain conditions. To illustrate, QST measures including pain threshold and conditioned pain modulation were recently shown to predict the efficacy of topical diclofenac sodium gel and pregabalin in patients with symptomatic knee osteoarthritis [25] and chronic pancreatitis [26], respectively.

Conclusion

This chapter briefly describes QST and its clinical relevance for chronic pain. However, it should be noted that the comprehensive measurement of pain experiences with QST generally requires costly equipment as well as methodologies that are technically elaborate and time consuming. This limits the clinical implementation of QST at present. However, there are ongoing efforts to develop QST procedures that are relatively brief, inexpensive, and require minimal technical expertise. Whether or not a simple collection of QST procedures could be routinely included in clinical practice and clinical trials focused on chronic pain is worthy of additional consideration.

References

1. Breivik H, Borchgrevink PC, Allen SM, Rosseland LA, Romundstad L, Hals EK, et al. Assessment of pain. Br J Anaesth. 2008;101(1):17–24.
2. Arendt-Nielsen L, Yarnitsky D. Experimental and clinical applications of quantitative sensory testing applied to skin, muscles and viscera. J Pain. 2009;10(6):556–72.
3. Cruz-Almeida Y, Fillingim RB. Can quantitative sensory testing move us closer to mechanism-based pain management? Pain Med. 2014;15(1):61–72.
4. Hansson P, Backonja M, Bouhassira D. Usefulness and limitations of quantitative sensory testing: clinical and research application in neuropathic pain states. Pain. 2007;129(3):256–9.
5. Pavlakovic G, Petzke F. The role of quantitative sensory testing in the evaluation of musculoskeletal pain conditions. Curr Rheumatol Rep. 2010;12(6):455–61.
6. Granovsky Y, Yarnitsky D. Personalized pain medicine: the clinical value of psychophysical assessment of pain modulation profile. Rambam Maimonides Med J. 2013;4(4):e0024.
7. Yarnitsky D, Granot M, Granovsky Y. Pain modulation profile and pain therapy: between pro- and antinociception. Pain. 2014;155(4):663–5.
8. Grosen K, Fischer IW, Olesen AE, Drewes AM. Can quantitative sensory testing predict responses to analgesic treatment? Eur J Pain. 2013;17(9):1267–80.
9. Olesen AE, Andresen T, Staahl C, Drewes AM. Human experimental pain models for assessing the therapeutic efficacy of analgesic drugs. Pharmacol Rev. 2012;64(3):722–79.
10. Eisenberg E, Midbari A, Haddad M, Pud D. Predicting the analgesic effect to oxycodone by 'static' and 'dynamic' quantitative sensory testing in healthy subjects. Pain. 2010;151(1):104–9.
11. Olesen SS, van Goor H, Bouwense SA, Wilder-Smith OH, Drewes AM. Reliability of static and dynamic quantitative sensory testing in patients with painful chronic pancreatitis. Reg Anesth Pain Med. 2012;37(5):530–6.
12. Nir RR, Yarnitsky D. Conditioned pain modulation. Curr Opin Support Palliat Care. 2015;9(2):131–7.

13. Sprenger C, Bingel U, Buchel C. Treating pain with pain: supraspinal mechanisms of endogenous analgesia elicited by heterotopic noxious conditioning stimulation. Pain. 2011;152(2):428–39.
14. Staud R, Vierck CJ, Cannon RL, Mauderli AP, Price DD. Abnormal sensitization and temporal summation of second pain (wind-up) in patients with fibromyalgia syndrome. Pain. 2001;91(1–2):165–75.
15. Staud R, Cannon RC, Mauderli AP, Robinson ME, Price DD, Vierck CJ Jr. Temporal summation of pain from mechanical stimulation of muscle tissue in normal controls and subjects with fibromyalgia syndrome. Pain. 2003;102(1–2):87–95.
16. Herrero JF, Laird JM, Lopez-Garcia JA. Wind-up of spinal cord neurones and pain sensation: much ado about something? Prog Neurobiol. 2000;61(2):169–203.
17. Edwards RR, Sarlani E, Wesselmann U, Fillingim RB. Quantitative assessment of experimental pain perception: multiple domains of clinical relevance. Pain. 2005;114(3):315–9.
18. Petersen KK, Arendt-Nielsen L, Simonsen O, Wilder-Smith O, Laursen MB. Presurgical assessment of temporal summation of pain predicts the development of chronic postoperative pain 12 months after total knee replacement. Pain. 2015;156(1):55–61.
19. Yarnitsky D, Crispel Y, Eisenberg E, Granovsky Y, Ben-Nun A, Sprecher E, et al. Prediction of chronic post-operative pain: pre-operative DNIC testing identifies patients at risk. Pain. 2008;138(1):22–8.
20. Valencia C, Fillingim RB, George SZ. Suprathreshold heat pain response is associated with clinical pain intensity for patients with shoulder pain. J Pain. 2011;12(1):133–40.
21. Goodin BR, Bulls HW, Herbert MS, Schmidt J, King CD, Glover TL, et al. Temporal summation of pain as a prospective predictor of clinical pain severity in adults aged 45 years and older with knee osteoarthritis: ethnic differences. Psychosom Med. 2014;76(4):302–10.
22. Edwards RR, Haythornthwaite JA, Tella P, Max MB, Raja S. Basal heat pain thresholds predict opioid analgesia in patients with postherpetic neuralgia. Anesthesiology. 2006;104(6):1243–8.
23. Yarnitsky D, Granot M, Nahman-Averbuch H, Khamaisi M, Granovsky Y. Conditioned pain modulation predicts duloxetine efficacy in painful diabetic neuropathy. Pain. 2012;153(6):1193–8.
24. Niesters M, Proto PL, Aarts L, Sarton EY, Drewes AM, Dahan A. Tapentadol potentiates descending pain inhibition in chronic pain patients with diabetic polyneuropathy. Br J Anaesth. 2014;113(1):148–56.
25. Edwards RR, Dolman AJ, Martel MO, Finan PH, Lazaridou A, Cornelius M, et al. Variability in conditioned pain modulation predicts response to NSAID treatment in patients with knee osteoarthritis. BMC Musculoskelet Disord. 2016;17:284.
26. Olesen SS, Graversen C, Bouwense SA, van Goor H, Wilder-Smith OH, Drewes AM. Quantitative sensory testing predicts pregabalin efficacy in painful chronic pancreatitis. PLoS One. 2013;8(3):e57963.

Part III

Cases

Case 1: High Dose Opioids and Multiple Pain Medications

11

Puneet Mishra and David A. Edwards

Considerations for Treatment of Acute on Chronic Pain

A patient with chronic pain who is admitted to the hospital with acute pain can pose challenges for attaining adequate pain control while balancing safety. There are three important considerations when developing a plan of treatment. First, in order to prevent suffering, a patient's baseline pain should be adequately treated. Second, additional treatments should be offered for acute pain. Finally, the treatment options should target the pain type and account for patient comorbidities as well as be designed to limit potential adverse effects.

High Dose Opioids

Opioid related adverse effects correlate with increasing dose. Some of these include sedation, respiratory depression, confusion, constipation, and urinary retention, as well as tolerance, dependence, and use disorders with long-term treatment. This patient is on both extended release and immediate release formulations of oxycodone for treatment of chronic low back pain. The morphine equivalent daily dose (MEDD) is 180 mg (see Chap. 28 for conversion table). This is considered a high dose with considerable risk for accidental overdose [1]. However, this patient may be tolerant to this dose and generally this should be continued during acute admission.

P. Mishra (✉)
Department of Anesthesiology, Vanderbilt University Medical Center, Nashville, TN, USA
e-mail: puneet.mishra@vumc.org

D. A. Edwards
Departments of Anesthesiology and Neurological Surgery, Vanderbilt University Medical Center, Nashville, TN, USA
e-mail: david.a.edwards@vumc.org

© Springer Nature Switzerland AG 2022
D. A. Edwards et al. (eds.), *Hospitalized Chronic Pain Patient*,
https://doi.org/10.1007/978-3-031-08376-1_11

Table 11.1 Conditions increasing risk for opioid related adverse events

Renal failure
- Opioids and non-opioid analgesics that depend on renal clearance may accumulate in the setting of acute renal failure (morphine, oxycodone, gabapentin, baclofen)

Obstructive sleep apnea
- Patients with OSA are at increased risk of accidental overdose death when treated with opioids and sedating combinations of medications (benzodiazepines)

Drug–drug interactions
- Medications used to treat other illnesses may alter the plasma concentration of opioids, increasing the risks (antibiotic or antipsychotic inhibitors of CYP450 enzymes raise plasma opioid levels)
- Benzodiazepine and opioid combinations significantly increase the risk of sedation and respiratory depression

Multimodal Analgesia

One way of improving this patient's pain control and limiting the need for excessive opioid dose escalation is to introduce multimodal analgesia (MMA). Multimodal analgesia is the use of pain treatments (both medication and non-medication) that target the pain type and that can be used to take advantage of their synergy and limit the need for high doses (and high frequency of side-effects) of any medication. This is in contrast to polypharmacy, which is the situation of multiple medications used at doses that increase the overall risk to a patient.

Co-Morbid Conditions and Risk of Overdose

Co-morbid conditions can result in tipping the balance of risk-benefit of opioids towards increased risk (Table 11.1). Extreme caution should be used when starting combinations of medications that may increase risk in certain patients, especially if continued after discharge. For example, initial chronic use of opioids and concurrent benzodiazepines increases the risk of opioid-related overdose fivefold [2].

References

1. Dunn KM, Saunders KW, Rutter CM, et al. Opioid prescriptions for chronic pain and overdose: a cohort study. Ann Intern Med. 2010;152:85–92.
2. Hernandez I, He M, Brooks MM, Zhang Y. Exposure-response association between concurrent opioid and benzodiazepine use and risk of opioid-related overdose in Medicare Part D beneficiaries. JAMA Netw Open. 2018;1(2):e180919.

Case 2: Buprenorphine

12

Rebecca Donald, Brandon Gish, Daniel Lonergan, and David A. Edwards

Key Points
- Determining mechanism, pharmacokinetics and dosing details of buprenorphine/ naloxone (Suboxone).
- Management of patients on buprenorphine based on the indication of their use (e.g. pain versus opioid use disorder).
- Treatment strategies using non-pharmacologic options for pain management in patients on buprenorphine.

Background

- Buprenorphine/naloxone is effective for the treatment of opioid use disorder (OUD) in an outpatient office-based setting (*Level 1*) [1].
- Buprenorphine/naloxone is effective in patients with chronic pain and opioid dependence (*Level 1*) [1].

R. Donald (✉)
Department of Anesthesiology, Vanderbilt University Medical Center, Nashville, TN, USA
e-mail: rebecca.donald@vumc.org

B. Gish
Commonwealth Pain and Spine, Nicholasville, KY, USA

D. Lonergan
Cuyuna Regional Medical Center, Crosby, MN, USA

D. A. Edwards
Departments of Anesthesiology and Neurological Surgery, Vanderbilt University Medical Center, Nashville, TN, USA
e-mail: david.a.edwards@vumc.org

© Springer Nature Switzerland AG 2022
D. A. Edwards et al. (eds.), *Hospitalized Chronic Pain Patient*,
https://doi.org/10.1007/978-3-031-08376-1_12

- To date there have been no randomized controlled studies published evaluating pain management modalities for patients maintained on buprenorphine treatment for addiction. Recommendations are based on pre-clinical data [2], case reports [3], and retrospective cohort studies [4, 5].

Pharmacology

Buprenorphine is considered a partial mu agonist which gives it a unique pharmacologic profile compared to full mu agonist opioids. As a partial mu agonist, buprenorphine binds to and activates the mu receptor, but it has lower intrinsic activity at the mu receptor compared to opioids that are considered full mu agonists. Buprenorphine still has the ability to provide potent analgesia, but it has a ceiling effect on euphoria, respiratory depression, sedation, and the development of physical dependence [6, 7] (Table 12.1). It is these latter qualities that make it safer than full mu opioid agonists. Despite this ceiling effect, the combination of buprenorphine with other non-opioid sedative drugs, such as benzodiazepines, can still result in overdose.

Buprenorphine has a very high affinity for the mu opioid receptor (Table 12.2) and a very slow dissociation from the opioid receptor with a half-life of approximately 37 h [8]. The high binding affinity for the mu opioid receptor means that

Table 12.1 Benefits and barriers of buprenorphine

Benefits	Barriers
• Reduces cravings for opioids • Mitigates withdrawal symptoms • Dampens euphoric effects of other opioids • Ceiling effect on respiratory depression and sedation • Long duration (37 h 1/2 life)	Potential to dampen analgesic effects of other opioids (depending on buprenorphine dose)

Table 12.2 Equilibrium dissociation constant (Ki value) of many opioids are reflective of receptor affinity (lower Ki value = greater mu receptor affinity)

	Ki value (nM)
Tramadol	12,486
Codeine	734.2
Meperidine	450.1
Hydrocodone	41.6
Oxycodone	25.9
Methadone	3.4
Fentanyl	1.35
Morphine	1.17
Oxymorphone	0.41
Hydromorphone	0.37
Buprenorphine	0.22
Sufentanil	0.14

buprenorphine not only prevents the binding of less potent opioids to the receptor, but also that it displaces other opioids from the receptor and can precipitate opioid withdrawal [1, 9].

Buprenorphine Formulations

Buprenorphine comes in formulations that are FDA approved for pain or FDA approved for the treatment of OUD (Fig. 12.1).

- Buprenorphine for pain comes in two forms: buccal and transdermal. Dosages are in micrograms/dose.
- Buprenorphine for OUD comes in a variety of forms including sublingual, buccal, and injectable. The implantable formulation, Probuphine, was withdrawn from the market in 2020. Doses of buprenorphine for OUD are much higher than those used for pain and are prescribed in milligrams/dose.
- Naloxone is added to many of these buprenorphine products as an abuse deterrent. For example, Suboxone is a combination medication that contains buprenorphine and naloxone in a 4:1 ratio. Naloxone is not absorbed well by either sublingual or oral routes of administration, so clinically significant opioid antagonism does not occur when these medications are used properly. If the medication is administered intravenously, however, the naloxone will have significant opioid antagonism, preventing the euphoric effects, and could precipitate symptoms of opioid withdrawal.
- In many states it is legal to use these high-dose formulations (commonly Suboxone) off-label to treat pain in patients who do not have OUD, while in other states it is not.

Buprenorphine formulations FDA approved for chronic pain

	Brand Name	Generic
FDA approved for Chronic Pain	Belbuca	buprenorphine buccal film (available doses: 75mcg –900mcg BID)
	Butrans	buprenorphine transdermal patch (available doses: 5, 7.5, 10, 15, 20 mcg/h)
	Norspan	buprenorphine transdermal patch (available doses: 5, 10, 20, 25, 30, 40 mcg/h)
	Buprenex	buprenorphine IV injection

Buprenorphine formulations FDA approved for opioid use disorder

	Brand Name	Generic
FDA Approved for Opioid Use Disorder	Bunavail	Buprenorphine naloxone buccal film
	Probuphine	buprenorphine intradermal implant (discontinued 10/20)
	Sublocade	buprenorphine extended-release subcutaneous injection
	Suboxone	Buprenorphine naloxone sublingual tablet or film
	Subutex	buprenorphine sublingual tablet
	Zubsolv	Buprenorphine naloxone sublingual tablet

Fig. 12.1 Buprenorphine formulations FDA-approved for the treatment of opioid use disorder

Buprenorphine Management for Surgery

When a patient is using buprenorphine for pain (μg doses), it is appropriate to continue their baseline dose of buprenorphine and supplement with multimodal adjuncts (Table 12.3) and full mu agonist opioids when necessary. This is because at microgram doses there are ample opioid receptors available for binding of full mu agonists.

Because of its unique pharmacodynamic properties, perioperative management of patients taking buprenorphine for OUD can be challenging. Research on the perioperative management of buprenorphine is ongoing, but it is now recommended that buprenorphine therapy be continued (although potentially at lower doses) in the perioperative period. Evidence has shown that pain can be adequately treated in the perioperative period while continuing buprenorphine, and the risks of discontinuing treatment likely outweigh any potential benefit [10, 11] (Table 12.4). This is because when buprenorphine is being prescribed for OUD, discontinuing it for surgery exposes patients to risk of withdrawal in the lead-up to surgery, difficulty resuming buprenorphine after surgery (re-induction), and potentially to periods of stress that may trigger lapse or relapse.

At doses of buprenorphine greater than 16 mg per day, opioid receptors are mostly saturated leaving very few receptors available for full mu agonist opioids (e.g., fentanyl, morphine, hydromorphone) to bind. Doses higher than 8 mg per day may continue to have clinically significant effects for over 72 h after the last dose, limiting the efficacy of other full agonist opioids during this period. Doses less than 8 mg per day may have less significant clinical consequences in the perioperative period, especially beyond 24 h after the last dose. In general, patients should be continued on buprenorphine (ideally 8 mg daily or less), and if pain control is not achieved after optimization of multimodal adjuncts, full mu agonist opioids can be added as necessary to achieve adequate analgesia. It is important to remember that because of the high binding affinity of buprenorphine to the mu opioid receptor, full mu agonist opioids will have significantly less analgesic effect upon administration, and higher doses of these agents may be required to out-compete buprenorphine for its position on the receptor. Ideally, patients should be discharged on buprenorphine (although not necessarily at their preoperative dose), and depending on their

Table 12.3 Multimodal analgesia non-opioid pain medicines

Drug	Route	Example dose and frequency
Acetaminophen	PO/IV	1000 mg q 8 h (more than 50 kg)
Ibuprofen	PO	600 mg q 6 h
Ketorolac	PO/IV	15–30 mg q 6 h
Celecoxib	PO	200–400 mg q 12 h
Gabapentin	PO	600–800 mg TID
Pregabalin	PO	75–150 mg q 12 h
Ketamine	IV	0.5 mg/kg bolus; infusion 0.25 mg/kg/h

Table 12.4 Guidelines for management of opioid agonists, mixed and partial agonists, and antagonists before surgery

Category		Mechanism	1/2 Life	Patient action plan
mu-opioid agonists/ opioid agonist abuse deterrent formulations	**Codeine** (many formulations, usually combined with acetaminophen or NSAID)	mu-agonist	3 h	Continue as prescribed (or reduce as tolerated)
	Fentanyl (Fentora, Actiq, OTFC, fentanyl patches)	mu-agonist	Dependent on formulation	
	Hydrocodone (Lortab, Vicodin, Zohydro, Hysingla)	mu-agonist	4 h	
	Hydromorphone (Dilaudid)	mu-agonist	2–3 h	
	Levorphanol	mu, delta, kappa-agonist, NMDA antagonist, SNRI	11–16 h	
	Meperidine (Demerol)	mu-agonist, K-agonist, DAT inhibitor, NE reuptake inhibitor	2.5–4 h	
	Methadone (Dolophine, Methadose)	mu-agonist, NMDA antagonist	8–59 h	
	Morphine (MS Contin, Oramorph)	mu-agonist	3–4 h (short-acting formulation); 11–13 h (long-acting formulation)	
	Morphine ER-naltrexone (Embeda)	(morphine) mu-agonist; (naltrexone) mu-antagonist inactive unless crushed	extended release dosed every 12–24 h	
	Oxycodone (Percocet, Roxicodone, OxyContin, Xtampza, Endocet, Roxicet, Percodan)	mu-agonist	Immediate release: 3–4 h; long-acting formations: 4.5–5.5 h	
	Oxycodone-naltrexone (Troxyca ER)	(oxycodone) mu-agonist; (naltrexone) mu-antagonist unless altered	7 h	
	Oxymorphone (Opana, Numorphan)	mu-agonist	Immediate release: 7–9 h; long-acting formulations: 9–11 h	

(continued)

Table 12.4 (continued)

Category		Mechanism	1/2 Life	Patient action plan
	Tapentadol (Nucynta)	mu-agonist, SNRI	Immediate release: 4 h; long-acting formulations 5–6 h	
	Tramadol (Ultram, Ultram ER)	mu-agonist, SNRI	Immediate release: 6–9 h; Extended release 8–11 h	
Mixed or partial opioid agonist/ antagonists	**Buprenorphine for OUD** • **Buprenorphine-naloxone** (Suboxone, Zubsolv, Bunavail) • **Buprenorphine** monoproduct (Subutex) • **Buprenorphine** extended-release administered as a monthly injection (Sublocade)	(Buprenorphine) mu-partial agonist, kappa-antagonist, delta-antagonist; (naloxone) mu-antagonist	37 h	Reduce dose to 8–16 mg on the day of surgery. Maintain on 4 mg BID during the acute post-operative period. Consider transitioning extended-release buprenorphine (Sublocade) to sublingual Suboxone and postponing elective surgery until the end of the dosing interval
	Buprenorphine for pain • **Belbuca** (buccal film) • **Norspan** (transdermal patch) • **Butrans** (transdermal patch) • **Buprenex** (IV, IM)	(Buprenorphine) mu-partial agonist, kappa-antagonist, delta-antagonist	Belbuca: 16–39 h; IV 2–3 h; transdermal patch 26 h	Continue sublingual and patch formulations throughout the perioperative period. Consider stopping Buprenex and replacing with a full mu agonist.
	Butorphanol (Stadol)	mu-partial agonist, K-partial agonist, delta-antagonist	2–9 h	Hold the morning of surgery
	Pentazocine (Talwin)	mu-antagonist, K-agonist, sigma-agonist	2–5 h	

Table 12.4 (continued)

Category		Mechanism	1/2 Life	Patient action plan
Opioid antagonists	**Bupropion-naltrexone** (Contrave)	(bupropion) NDRI, nicotine receptor antagonist; (naltrexone) mu-antagonist	4 h	Stop Contrave 24 h before surgery, continue bupropion during perioperative period, reinitiate Contrave 7 days after cessation of post-operative opioid therapy
	Naltrexone (Vivitrol, ReVia, Depade)	mu-antagonist	4–13 h Depot injection lasts approx. 1 month	Hold 72 h before surgery unless long acting depot version (Vivitrol). This needs to be held 28–31 days before surgery. Must be off opioids before restarting postoperatively
	Naloxone (Narcan, Evzio)	mu-antagonist	0.5–1.5 h	Hold the morning of surgery. Must be off opioids before restarting postoperatively
	Nalbuphine (Nubain)	mu-antagonist, K-agonist	5 h	
	Methylnaltrexone (Relistor)	mu-antagonist (peripherally acting)	15 h	Continue
	Naloxegol (Movantik, Moventig)	mu-antagonist (peripherally acting)	6–11 h	

[a] Filled boxes—recommended preoperative specialist consultation for perioperative management protocol

analgesic requirement, they may also need to be discharged on a full mu agonist opioid with a plan to taper the full mu agonist and return to their preoperative dose of buprenorphine when the acute pain improves [11].

It is important to seek out non-opioid, multi-disciplinary methods of pain control in all patients, especially those on buprenorphine maintenance therapy. It is generally a good strategy to combine multimodal analgesics (Table 12.3) with regional and neuraxial anesthesia where possible. If opioids are required in a patient with recent buprenorphine use, carefully titrate doses to effect, and expect that these may be higher than typical doses.

Regional and Neuraxial Anesthesia

In the presence or absence of buprenorphine, regional anesthesia and neuraxial anesthetic techniques can provide significant pain control during the immediate postoperative period. This is particularly true for procedures on the limbs which are easily amenable to single shot or continuous peripheral nerve blockade. The expected duration of pain and the available options for regional anesthesia should be evaluated before deciding whether to dose-reduce a patient's buprenorphine perioperatively.

Option 1: Elective Surgery: Continue Buprenorphine Therapy, Consider Dose Reduction

- For elective surgery, in patients taking >16 mg/day of buprenorphine/naloxone, maintain the patient's current dose until the day before surgery. On the day before surgery reduce the dose to 8–16 mg/day. On the day of surgery and on subsequent post-operative days the patient should receive 8 mg daily, ideally dosed as 4 mg BID. Optimize pain control with multimodal analgesics and regional/neuraxial anesthesia. If additional opioids are ultimately required, short-acting, high affinity full agonists (e.g., hydromorphone, fentanyl) may be used. These doses may be higher than normally expected, and thus appropriate monitoring must be available. When severe post-operative pain has resolved, the full mu agonist can be tapered, and the patient can resume their original dose of buprenorphine/naloxone [12].

Option 2: Urgent/Unexpected Surgery: Use Clinical Judgment

- When confronted with an unplanned surgery or trauma in a patient on buprenorphine/naloxone, begin treatment with a multimodal regimen and use clinical judgment to determine the benefits of continuation of buprenorphine/naloxone at current dose versus dose-reduction.
- A person with a short recovery period may be easily managed by continuing the buprenorphine/naloxone as prescribed (possibly in divided doses q6–8 h) and using additional opioid agonists for pain control.
- A person with a prolonged recovery may benefit from buprenorphine at a reduced dose (4 mg BID) with the addition of full mu agonists.
- Be cautious when combining high-dose buprenorphine with high-dose full mu agonists as there is risk for sedation and respiratory depression. Close monitoring should be available and ICU admission may be indicated.
- Attempts should be made to resume the patient on their home buprenorphine/naloxone regimen prior to discharge. When this is not possible, a very short course of opioids may be considered. This should be done only in conjunction with close follow up for treatment of addiction and a clear plan for resuming the patient's full dose of buprenorphine/naloxone.

Case Discussion

In the above case, the expected length of stay is likely only a few days. The patient's total daily buprenorphine/naloxone dose is 16/4 mg, of which his last dose of 8/2 mg was this morning. He could continue buprenorphine 8 mg daily (dosed 4 mg BID) during the acute post-operative period with the addition of multimodal analgesics, such as acetaminophen 1 g PO, ketorolac 30 mg IV, and gabapentin 600 mg PO. If additional analgesia is needed a full mu agonist such as hydromorphone or fentanyl could be added as necessary to provide adequate analgesia.

If the patient has no apparent contraindication to regional anesthesia, a preoperatively placed supraclavicular perineural catheter could provide excellent analgesia for the post-operative period. This would allow him to continue buprenorphine/naloxone at his baseline dose and likely would obviate the need for additional full mu agonists opioids to be used.

Upon discharge planning it is important that follow up be arranged with the patient's buprenorphine/naloxone prescriber.

References

1. Chen KY, Chen L, Mao J. Buprenorphine–naloxone therapy in pain management. Anesthesiology. 2014;120(5):1262–74.
2. Kögel B, Christoph T, Strassburger W, Friderichs E. Interaction of mu-opioid receptor agonists and antagonists with the analgesic effect of buprenorphine in mice. Eur J Pain. 2005;9(5):599–611.
3. Kornfeld H, Manfredi L. Effectiveness of full agonist opioids in patients stabilized on buprenorphine undergoing major surgery: a case series. Am J Ther. 2010;17(5):523–8.
4. Li AH, Schmiesing C, Aggarwal AK. Evidence for continuing buprenorphine in the perioperative period. Clin J Pain. 2020;36(10):764–74.
5. Quaye A, Potter K, Roth S, Acampora G, Mao J, Zhang Y. Perioperative continuation of buprenorphine at low-moderate doses was associated with lower postoperative pain scores and decreased outpatient opioid dispensing compared with buprenorphine discontinuation. Pain Med. 2020;21(9):1955–60.
6. Gudin J, Fudin J. A narrative pharmacological review of buprenorphine: a unique opioid for the treatment of chronic pain. Pain Ther. 2020;9(1):41–54. https://doi.org/10.1007/s40122-019-00143-6.
7. Schuh KJ, Walsh SL, Stitzer ML. Onset, magnitude, and duration of opioid blockade produced by buprenorphine and naltrexone in humans. Psychopharmacology (Berl). 1999;145(2):162–14.
8. Sen S, et al. New pain management options for the surgical patient on methadone and buprenorphine. Curr Pain Headache Rep. 2016;20(3):16.
9. Volpe DA, McMahon Tobin GA, Mellon RD, Katki AG, Parker RJ, Colatsky T, Kropp TJ, Verbois SL. Uniform assessment and ranking of opioid μ receptor binding constants for selected opioid drugs. Regul Toxicol Pharmacol. 2011;59(3):385–90.
10. Edwards DA, Hedrick TL, Jayaram J, Argoff C, Gulur P, Holubar SD, Gan TJ, Mythen MG, Miller TE, Shaw AD, Thacker JKM, McEvoy MD. American society for enhanced recovery and perioperative quality initiative joint consensus statement on perioperative management of patients on preoperative opioid therapy. Anesth Analg. 2019;129(2):553–66.

11. Goel A, Azargive S, Weissman JS, Shanthanna H, Hanlon JG, Samman B, Dominicis M, et al. Perioperative Pain and Addiction Interdisciplinary Network (Pain) Clinical Practice Advisory for perioperative management of buprenorphine: results of a modified Delphi process. Br J Anaesth. 2019;123(2):e333–e42.
12. Acampora GA. Special issues for patients with SUDs undergoing surgery. Psychiatr Times. 2020;37(5):97.

Case 3: Methadone

Puneet Mishra and David A. Edwards

Pharmacology

Methadone is a synthetic opioid that acts at μ- and δ-opioid receptors and at the *N*-methyl-D-aspartate (NMDA) receptor to reduce pain [1]. The peak effect of oral methadone occurs at 3–4 h and of intravenous methadone at 8 min [2–4]. Methadone exists as two isomers, L-methadone and D-methadone, with L-methadone being up to 50 times more potent [5, 6]. Methadone is 86% protein bound and depends on CYPP450 3A4 (major) and 1A2 and 2D6 (minor) for metabolism (Table 13.1) [7, 8]. Its plasma concentrations can be significantly impacted by changes in protein level and by drug–drug interactions. Methadone is cleared fecally. It does not accumulate in renal failure and is poorly removed by dialysis. The duration of analgesia is 6–8 h, correlating with its α-elimination and has a subanalgesic persistence of up to 60 h correlating with β-elimination [9]. The complex pharmacology of methadone result in non-linear morphine equivalents, so caution must be used when converting [10] (Tables 13.2 and 13.3).

Methadone Indications

The properties of methadone make it useful for the treatment of acute pain, chronic pain, and opioid use disorder. Given its complexities it is best left to those with experience in managing these conditions safely with methadone. The rapid onset

P. Mishra (✉)
Department of Anesthesiology, Vanderbilt University Medical Center, Nashville, TN, USA
e-mail: puneet.mishra@vumc.org

D. A. Edwards
Departments of Anesthesiology and Neurological Surgery, Vanderbilt University Medical Center, Nashville, TN, USA
e-mail: david.a.edwards@vumc.org

© Springer Nature Switzerland AG 2022
D. A. Edwards et al. (eds.), *Hospitalized Chronic Pain Patient*,
https://doi.org/10.1007/978-3-031-08376-1_13

Table 13.1 Hepatic metabolism P450 and methadone

CYP P450 3A4 inducers (decrease methadone blood levels)	CYP P450 3A4 inhibitors (increased methadone blood levels)
Barbiturates	Cimetidine
Carbamazepine	Fluconazole
Oxcarbazepine	Itraconazole
Phenytoin	Ketoconazole
Topiramate	Erythromycin
Risperidone	Clarithromycin
Dexamethasone	Ritonavir[a]
	Nelfinavir[a]
	Diltiazem
	Verapamil
	Amiodarone
	Paroxetine
	Fluoxetine
	Venlafaxine
	Sertraline

[a]Despite CYP3A4 inhibition, methadone levels are decreased due to increased hepatic extraction and systemic metabolism induced by these drugs

Table 13.2 Conversion to methadone

Morphine milligram equivalent	Methadone
1–30	× 1/2
31–99	× 1/4
100–299	× 1/8
300–499	× 1/12
500–999	× 1/15
1000–1200	× 1/20
>1200	

Table 13.3 Methadone to morphine conversion

Methadone dose (mg/day)	
1–20	× 4
21–40	× 8
41–60	× 10
61–80	× 12

and long-duration make it useful for treatment of postoperative pain. Its action at μ-opioid and NMDA receptors with prolonged half-life make it useful in treatment of chronic severe pain. The long β-elimination prevent withdrawal but without causing euphoria, making it useful for the treatment of opioid use disorder.

Methadone and QTc

Methadone prolongs the QTc interval as measured on the electrocardiogram (ECG) and can result in arrhythmias (e.g., Torsades de pointes usually occurring at QTc >500 ms but with increased risk when >450 ms) [8]. This is more likely to occur when combined with other medications that also prolong the QTc (Table 13.4).

Table 13.4 Risk factors for prolonged QTc to consider when using methadone

- Electrolyte abnormalities (hypokalemia, hypomagnesemia)
- Impaired liver function
- Structural heart disease
- Congenital prolonged QTc
- Drugs that prolong QTc (clarithromycin, erythromycin, quetiapine, TCAs)
- Ethanol

When initiating methadone, it is recommended to first obtain an ECG to evaluate the QTc duration. It is recommended to use alternatives to methadone on patients with QTc >450 ms. When adjusting methadone, periodically check Qtc and consider reducing the dose if QTc >450 ms.

References

1. Ferrari A, Coccia CP, Bertolini A, Sternieri E. Methadone—metabolism, pharmacokinetics and interactions. Pharmacol Res. 2004;50(6):551–9.
2. Kharasch ED. Intraoperative methadone: rediscovery, reappraisal, and reinvigoration? Anesth Analg. 2011;112(1):13–6.
3. Nicholson AB, Watson GR, Derry S, Wiffen PJ. Methadone for cancer pain. Cochrane Database Syst Rev. 2017;2(2):CD003971.
4. Kharasch ED, Walker A, Whittington D, Hoffer C, Bedynek PS. Methadone metabolism and clearance are induced by nelfinavir despite inhibition of cytochrome P4503A (CYP3A) activity. Drug Alcohol Depend. 2009;101(3):158–68.
5. Fainsinger R, Schoeller T, Bruera E. Methadone in the management of cancer pain: a review. Pain. 1993;51(2):137–47.
6. Bruera E, Sweeney C. Methadone use in cancer patients with pain: a review. J Palliat Med. 2002;5(1):127–38.
7. Vieweg WV, Lipps WF, Fernandez A. Opioids and methadone equivalents for clinicians. Prim Care Companion J Clin Psychiatry. 2005;7(3):86–8.
8. Chou R, Cruciani RA, Fiellin DA, Compton P, Farrar JT, Haigney MC, Inturrisi C, Knight JR, Otis-Green S, Marcus SM, Mehta D, Meyer MC, Portenoy R, Savage S, Strain E, Walsh S, Zeltzer L, American Pain Society; Heart Rhythm Society. Methadone safety: a clinical practice guideline from the American Pain Society and College on Problems of Drug Dependence, in collaboration with the Heart Rhythm Society. J Pain. 2014;15(4):321–37.
9. Peng PW, Tumber PS, Gourlay D. Review article: perioperative pain management of patients on methadone therapy. Can J Anaesth. 2005;52(5):513–23.
10. Centers for Disease Control and Prevention. Calculating total daily dose of opioids for safer dosage. 2020. https://www.cdc.gov/drugoverdose/pdf/calculating_total_daily_dose-a.pdf.

Case 4: Abdominal Pain

Andrew J. B. Pisansky and Puneet Mishra

Abdominal Wall Pain

It is important to consider abdominal wall pain as an etiology as this pain generator is often overlooked and presents an opportunity for therapeutic intervention. Estimates vary by population, but the prevalence of abdominal wall pain among patients in whom diagnostic work up has been unrevealing may be as high as 15–30% [1]. The pain-signaling nerve fibers involved in abdominal wall pain are the cutaneous sensory nerve branches arising from the T7 to T12 dorsal rami and intercostal nerves. Entrapment or neuralgia of these nerves at or near their anterior insertion through the lateral border of the rectus sheath may produce anterior cutaneous nerve entrapment syndrome (ACNES) thus leading to abdominal wall pain. Similarly, abdominal wall neuralgia may present at sites of prior surgical incision. Physical examination may reveal a patient who is able to precisely localize the area of maximal discomfort with abdominal muscle contraction (e.g., Carnett's sign) [2].

In a patient who meets the clinical criteria for abdominal wall pain and lacks red flag symptoms (e.g., history of gastrointestinal bleeding, abnormal laboratory markers suggesting abdominal organ dysfunction, abdominal mass, or constitutional symptoms) a trigger point injection may be indicated for diagnostic confirmation and therapeutic management. Treatment typically begins with a diagnostic injection of local anesthetic and steroid to the point of maximal tenderness although other procedures such as transversus abdominal plane block (TAP) or rectus sheath block may also be considered.

Among a group of patients who meet the criteria for abdominal wall pain (e.g., localized abdominal wall pain with point of tenderness size <2.5 cm and positive Carnett's sign), 77% received complete relief from localized trigger point injection at an average follow up of 25 months [3]. This effect has been shown to be related

A. J. B. Pisansky (✉) · P. Mishra
Department of Anesthesiology, Vanderbilt University Medical Center, Nashville, TN, USA
e-mail: andrew.pisansky@vumc.org; puneet.mishra@vumc.org

© Springer Nature Switzerland AG 2022
D. A. Edwards et al. (eds.), *Hospitalized Chronic Pain Patient*,
https://doi.org/10.1007/978-3-031-08376-1_14

to local anesthetic rather than needling or volume effects and repeat injection is often necessary [4, 5]. Additional therapies for patients who do not respond to local trigger point injection but have abdominal wall pain include pulsed radiofrequency, surgical release, and chemical neurolysis. There are no established medical therapies for this condition, though standard medical interventions for peripheral neuralgia may be appropriate for trial in refractory cases for whom other interventional techniques are not acceptable or are contraindicated.

Chronic Pancreatitis

Chronic pancreatitis can be due to numerous causes and often is relapsing and only incompletely remitting. Chronic pancreatitis may mimic other disease states of nearby organs (e.g., abdominal vascular disease; disease of other abdominal viscera) and over time, patients with chronic pancreatitis may be at increased risk for pancreatic cancer. Thus, treating physicians must remain vigilant to other causes for abdominal pain that may be life threatening, particularly in this population.

The natural history of chronic pancreatitis is variable, but in many cases, patients continue to have episodic abdominal pain despite ongoing medical management. Conservative therapies include dietary and lifestyle modification (e.g. abstinence from alcohol and smoking, medium chain fatty acid diet, pancreatic enzyme supplementation, and antioxidant supplements) [6].

Over time, continued inflammation often leads to visceral hypersensitivity which coexists with the acute inflammation during acute pancreatitis pain flares [7]. The mechanisms of pain are both peripheral and central and cohorts examining the results of interventional therapy in chronic pancreatitis have shown that a minority of patients respond positively to diagnostic injection of visceral afferent nerve fibers [8].

Clinical trials studying non-opioid medications for treatment of pain related to chronic pancreatitis are limited. In a randomized controlled trial among patients with chronic pancreatitis, pregabalin was found to be superior to placebo as an adjunctive pain control medication [9]. Centrally acting agents such as the tricyclic antidepressants (TCAs) amitriptyline and nortriptyline have been found to be effective in neuropathic pain conditions, but there is limited support for these agents in the treatment of chronic pancreatitis and recommendations for use of these agents are largely extrapolated from the few positive trials in other cases of visceral hypersensitivity (see below under inflammatory bowel disease).

Opioid use may theoretically cause sphincter of Oddi spasm and preclinical data suggest that use of mu-opioid receptor agonists may worsen acute episodes of pancreatitis via mechanisms other than worsened sphincter or Oddi dysfunction including delayed inflammatory resolution and pancreatic regeneration [10]. Despite these caveats, most patients who are hospitalized for an acute flare of pancreatitis require opioids during hospitalization and cross-sectional data suggest that approximately 80% of patients will receive opioids during admission for pancreatitis [11].

Interventional procedures include percutaneous and endoscopic celiac plexus block. In a small randomized controlled trial (N = 22) of endoscopic ultrasound guided versus computed tomography (CT) guided celiac plexus block, higher rates of pain reduction were observed with endoscopic as compared to CT-guided celiac plexus block [12]. Outcomes in a larger follow up trial of 90 patients conducted by the same authors reported mean pain score decrease from 8 to 2 on a visual analog scale at 4 and 8 weeks. Over time, the percentage of patients who continued to derive benefit decreased to 26% at 12 weeks and 10% at 24 weeks [13].

For patients who do not obtain sustained benefit from celiac plexus block and who are not candidates for surgery, spinal cord stimulation (SCS) is also an option. In a retrospective study of 24 patients with chronic pancreatitis, SCS lead placement at the T5 or T6 level was associated with an average VAS score of 3.6 at one year follow up, improved from an average VAS score of 8 prior to SCS trial [14].

Surgical management includes endoscopic relief of the pancreatic duct, and surgical decompression or resection, though the results of these interventions have shown mixed results and are associated with increased morbidity compared to less invasive interventions.

Inflammatory Bowel Disease

Inflammatory bowel disease (IBD) includes Crohn's disease and ulcerative colitis, both of which involve inflammatory changes to the intestinal wall, principally involve ileum, colon, and rectum. Pain related to these disorders may be due to acute inflammation or sequelae from disease such as stricture formation resulting in bowel obstruction.

First line therapies for patients with IBD are targeted at the underlying disease process by use of disease modifying therapeutics targeting the resolution of inflammatory changes to the bowel wall and mucosa. Outpatient strategies include dietary modification focused on avoidance of short chain carbohydrates, which tend to worsen functional symptoms of bloating, gas pains, and diarrhea. In patients who have diarrheal symptoms without active signs of mucosal inflammation, an antidiarrheal such as loperamide may be employed, but these are rarely continued in the hospitalized patient or the patient with signs of active inflammation.

Options for medical management of abdominal pain are guided more by the individual patient situation. For instance, the use of tricyclic antidepressants may be preferable in the patient with diarrheal symptoms due to the anticholinergic effects of this class; similarly, they may be avoided in patients who have predominantly constipation. Much of the data for management of the functional symptoms associated with IBD (e.g., pain, spasms) are guided by literature related to irritable bowel syndrome (IBS). Use of antispasmodics has been shown in meta-analysis to provide relief of abdominal pain [15]. Among these, the most commonly used agents are hyoscyamine and dicyclomine. When there is an element of severe abdominal wall spasm suspected, a trial of methocarbamol may be given intravenously, though there is only anecdotal evidence to support this approach.

Use of centrally acting neuropathic agents has been shown to be effective, with TCAs (imipramine, desipramine, and amitriptyline) showing positive data in meta-analysis of available trials [16]. Gabapentin has been shown in preclinical studies to decrease markers of intestinal inflammation, though there have been no definitive clinical trials to support its use for abdominal pain [17].

Use of interventional therapies is not supported in literature through rigorous study. There are case reports of spinal cord stimulation being used in patients with history of irritable bowel syndrome [18]. Intravenous lidocaine or intravenous ketamine is often used for inpatients with abdominal pain, but evidence for this indication is anecdotal [19].

Opioids are useful for severe acute pain uncontrolled by non-opioid analgesic methods. Use of opioids in hospitalized patients with acute on chronic abdominal pain must be balanced against the risks of escalating chronic doses, worsened bowel motility, constipation, and nausea.

Gastroparesis

Gastroparesis may have many causes, including diabetes, surgery, medication effects, neurological disease, or other factors. Common symptoms include pain, nausea, vomiting, postprandial discomfort, and bloating. First line therapies include prokinetic agents such as metoclopramide, domperidone, erythromycin and other macrolide antibiotics [20].

Treatment of refractory pain in gastroparesis has proven difficult, with limited studies showing mixed and unpromising results. Following positive trials for use of TCA's in functional symptoms of IBD and IBS, open label trials were conducted using a variety of TCAs for treatment of functional nausea and vomiting and reported positive results [21]. However, in a later randomized controlled trial examining the effect of nortriptyline on a combined score of gastroparetic symptoms, there was no effect over placebo [22]. Amitriptyline, however, was shown in a randomized trial to provide superior relief of painful dyspepsia (the specific symptom of uncomfortable abdominal fullness associated with gastroparesis) as compared to both placebo and escitalopram, a serotonin norepinephrine reuptake inhibitor [23]. Mirtazepine, an atypical antidepressant, has been shown to be efficacious for nausea, vomiting, and retching in a prospective cohort without comparator group, though there was no significant effect on upper abdominal pain [24].

There are no evidence-based interventional therapies for gastroparesis. Endoscopic intrapyloric injection of botulinum A toxin to the pyloric sphincter has been attempted, but data do not support its use [25].

References

1. Srinivasan R, Greenbaum DS. Chronic abdominal wall pain: a frequently overlooked problem. Practical approach to diagnosis and management. Am J Gastroenterol. 2002;97(4):824–30. https://doi.org/10.1111/j.1572-0241.2002.05662.x.
2. Koop H, Koprdova S, Schürmann C. Chronic abdominal wall pain. Dtsch Arztebl Int. 2016;113(4):51–7. https://doi.org/10.3238/arztebl.2016.0051.
3. Nazareno J, Ponich T, Gregor J. Long-term follow-up of trigger point injections for abdominal wall pain. Can J Gastroenterol. 2005;19(9):561–5. https://doi.org/10.1155/2005/274181.

4. Boelens OB, Scheltinga MR, Houterman S, Roumen RM. Randomized clinical trial of trigger point infiltration with lidocaine to diagnose anterior cutaneous nerve entrapment syndrome. Br J Surg. 2013;100(2):217–21. https://doi.org/10.1002/bjs.8958.
5. Greenbaum DS, Greenbaum RB, Joseph JG, Natale JE. Chronic abdominal wall pain. Diagnostic validity and costs. Dig Dis Sci. 1994;39(9):1935–41. https://doi.org/10.1007/bf02088128.
6. Singh VK, Yadav D, Garg PK. Diagnosis and management of chronic pancreatitis: a review. JAMA. 2019;322(24):2422–34. https://doi.org/10.1001/jama.2019.19411.
7. Buscher HC, Wilder-Smith OH, van Goor H. Chronic pancreatitis patients show hyperalgesia of central origin: a pilot study. Eur J Pain. 2006;10(4):363–70.
8. Conwell DL, Vargo JJ, Zuccaro G, Dews TE, Mekhail N, Scheman J, Shay SS. Role of differential neuroaxial blockade in the evaluation and management of pain in chronic pancreatitis. Am J Gastroenterol. 2001;96(2):431–6.
9. Olesen SS, Bouwense SA, Wilder-Smith OH, van Goor H, Drewes AM. Pregabalin reduces pain in patients with chronic pancreatitis in a randomized, controlled trial. Gastroenterology. 2011;141(2):536–43. https://doi.org/10.1053/j.gastro.2011.04.003.
10. Barlass U, Dutta R, Cheema H, George J, Sareen A, Dixit A, Saluja AK. Morphine worsens the severity and prevents pancreatic regeneration in mouse models of acute pancreatitis. Gut. 2018;67(4):600–2. https://doi.org/10.1136/gutjnl-2017-313717.
11. Wu BU, Butler RK, Chen W. Factors associated with opioid use in patients hospitalized for acute pancreatitis. JAMA Netw Open. 2019;2(4):e191827. https://doi.org/10.1001/jamanetworkopen.2019.1827.
12. Gress F, Schmitt C, Sherman S, Ikenberry S, Lehman G. A prospective randomized comparison of endoscopic ultrasound- and computed tomography-guided celiac plexus block for managing chronic pancreatitis pain. Am J Gastroenterol. 1999;94(4):900–5. https://doi.org/10.1111/j.1572-0241.1999.01042.x.
13. Gress F, Schmitt C, Sherman S, Ciaccia D, Ikenberry S, Lehman G. Endoscopic ultrasound-guided celiac plexus block for managing abdominal pain associated with chronic pancreatitis: a prospective single center experience. Am J Gastroenterol. 2001;96(2):409–16. https://doi.org/10.1111/j.1572-0241.2001.03551.x.
14. Kapural L, Cywinski JB, Sparks DA. Spinal cord stimulation for visceral pain from chronic pancreatitis. Neuromodul Technol Neural Interface. 2011;14(5):423–7.
15. Ruepert L, Quartero AO, de Wit NJ, van der Heijden GJ, Rubin G, Muris JW. Bulking agents, antispasmodics and antidepressants for the treatment of irritable bowel syndrome. Cochrane Database Syst Rev. 2011;8:Cd003460. https://doi.org/10.1002/14651858.CD003460.pub3.
16. Xie C, Tang Y, Wang Y, Yu T, Wang Y, Jiang L, Lin L. Efficacy and safety of antidepressants for the treatment of irritable bowel syndrome: a meta-analysis. PLoS One. 2015;10(8):e0127815. https://doi.org/10.1371/journal.pone.0127815.
17. de Brito TV, Júnior GJD, da Cruz Júnior JS, Silva RO, da Silva Monteiro CE, Franco AX, Barbosa A. Gabapentin attenuates intestinal inflammation: role of PPAR-gamma receptor. Eur J Pharmacol. 2020;873:172974. https://doi.org/10.1016/j.ejphar.2020.172974.
18. Krames E, Mousad DG. Spinal cord stimulation reverses pain and diarrheal episodes of irritable bowel syndrome: a case report. Neuromodul Technol Neural Interface. 2004;7(2):82–8.
19. Weibel S, Jelting Y, Pace NL, Helf A, Eberhart LH, Hahnenkamp K, Kranke P. Continuous intravenous perioperative lidocaine infusion for postoperative pain and recovery in adults. Cochrane Database Syst Rev. 2018;6:CD009642.
20. Camilleri M, Chedid V, Ford AC, Haruma K, Horowitz M, Jones KL, Stanghellini V. Gastroparesis. Nat Rev Dis Primers. 2018;4(1):41. https://doi.org/10.1038/s41572-018-0038-z.
21. Prakash C, Lustman PJ, Freedland KE, Clouse RE. Tricyclic antidepressants for functional nausea and vomiting: clinical outcome in 37 patients. Dig Dis Sci. 1998;43(9):1951–6. https://doi.org/10.1023/a:1018878324327.
22. Parkman HP, Van Natta ML, Abell TL, McCallum RW, Sarosiek I, Nguyen L, Pasricha PJ. Effect of nortriptyline on symptoms of idiopathic gastroparesis: the NORIG randomized clinical trial. JAMA. 2013;310(24):2640–9. https://doi.org/10.1001/jama.2013.282833.

23. Talley NJ, Locke GR, Saito YA, Almazar AE, Bouras EP, Howden CW, Zinsmeister AR. Effect of amitriptyline and escitalopram on functional dyspepsia: a multicenter randomized controlled study. Gastroenterology. 2015;149(2):340–9. https://doi.org/10.1053/j.gastro.2015.04.020.
24. Malamood M, Roberts A, Kataria R, Parkman HP, Schey R. Mirtazapine for symptom control in refractory gastroparesis. Drug Des Dev Ther. 2017;11:1035–41. https://doi.org/10.2147/dddt.S125743.
25. Bai Y, Xu M-J, Yang X, Xu C, Gao J, Zou D-W, Li Z-S. A systematic review on intrapyloric botulinum toxin injection for gastroparesis. Digestion. 2010;81(1):27–34.

Case 5: Unknown Pain Source

15

Jenna L. Walters

Fibromyalgia

Fibromyalgia is currently defined as pain elicited at 11 of 18 specific muscle and tendon points located bilaterally, above and below the waist. Patients also frequently exhibit alterations in concentration, mood and sleep patterns. Current diagnostic recommendations include obtaining a complete blood count, erythrocyte sedimentation rate, muscle enzymes, liver and thyroid function studies to rule out other systemic illnesses. There is a growing body of evidence supporting the association of fibromyalgia with psychiatric diagnoses such as anxiety and depression and other widespread painful syndromes such as rheumatological diseases, chronic pelvic and functional abdominal pain, temporomandibular joint disease and chronic tension headaches [1].

Conservative and Alternative Management

Strong evidence exists for establishing a regular exercise program. Additional alternative therapies based on availability include trigger point injections, physical therapy, massage therapy and possibly acupuncture [1, 2].

Pharmacologic Management

There are several analgesics that can be beneficial in the treatment of fibromyalgia pain (Table 15.1). These are most effective when used in combination with non-pharmacologic interventions and when they target the type of pain that is present.

J. L. Walters (✉)
Midlands Orthopaedics and Neurosurgery, Columbia, SC, USA

© Springer Nature Switzerland AG 2022
D. A. Edwards et al. (eds.), *Hospitalized Chronic Pain Patient*,
https://doi.org/10.1007/978-3-031-08376-1_15

Table 15.1 Pharmacologic treatment options, mechanisms of action and associated side effects for fibromyalgia

Medication	Mechanism of action	Side effects
Anticonvulsants 1. Gabapentin 2. Pregabalin	Block calcium channels	Dizziness, sedation, ataxia, peripheral edema, vision changes, weight gain, depression, Stevens–Johnson syndrome
SNRIs 1. Duloxetine 2. Milnacipran 3. Venlafaxine	Increase serotonin and norepinephrine to augment descending pain pathways	Nausea, headache, GI upset, decreased libido, blurred vision, weight changes, suicidality, serotonin syndrome, hepatotoxicity
Tricyclics 1. Nortriptyline 2. Amitriptyline	– Increase serotonin and norepinephrine to augment descending pain pathways – Block sodium channels – NMDA antagonist	Drowsiness, dizziness, palpitations, diaphoresis, orthostasis, seizure, extrapyramidal side effects, anti-cholinergic side effects, QT prolongation, suicidality
Muscle relaxants 1. Cyclobenzaprine	Increase norepinephrine in locus coeruleus	Drowsiness, dizziness, confusion, GI upset, anti-cholinergic side effects, arrhythmia, seizure
Local anesthetics 1. Lidocaine Infusion 5 mg/kg	Block sodium channels	Tremor, confusion, tinnitus, lethargy, arrhythmia, seizure, cardiovascular collapse
NMDA antagonists 1. Ketamine Infusion 0.3–0.5 mg/kg	Block NMDA receptor decreasing release of glutamate at the dorsal horn of the spinal cord	GI upset, BP and HR elevation, diplopia, hallucinations, respiratory depression, increased ICP
Non-steroidal anti-inflammatories	Inhibits cyclooxygenase, decreases prostaglandin and thromboxane	GI upset, GI bleeding, ash, hypertension, MI, nephrotoxicity, thrombocytopenia, Stevens–Johnson syndrome

Temporomandibular Joint Disorder

Temporomandibular disorders (TMDs) include painful conditions that involve the muscles of mastication and abnormalities in the temporomandibular joint. Deterioration within the joint produces an inflammatory process activating C-fibers and eventually leading to symptoms of peripheral sensitization. Similar to other functional pain syndromes, the development of central sensitization is believed to be associated with increases in intracellular calcium and activation of NMDA receptors within the dorsal horn of the spinal cord [3].

Conservative Management

Patients should be educated on muscle training and relaxation techniques along with utilization of an occlusal appliance. Additional conservative therapies include massage and transcutaneous electrical nerve stimulation (TENS) application [3].

Table 15.2 Pharmacologic treatment options, mechanisms of action and associated side effects for TMD

Medications	Mechanism of action	Side effects
Acetaminophen	Unknown	Nausea, rash, hepatotoxicity
Non-steroidal anti-inflammatories	Inhibits cyclooxygenase, decreases prostaglandin and thromboxane	GI upset, GI bleeding, ash, hypertension, MI, nephrotoxicity, thrombocytopenia, Stevens–Johnson syndrome
Muscle relaxants 1. Cyclobenzaprine 2. Tizanidine 3. Metaxalone 4. Methocarbamol	Exact mechanism unknown	Dizziness, sedation, confusion, GI upset, anti-cholinergic side effects, hypotension, arrhythmia
Tricyclic anti-depressants 1. Nortriptyline 2. Amitriptyline	1. Increase serotonin and norepinephrine to augment descending pain pathways 2. Block sodium channels 3. NMDA antagonist	Drowsiness, dizziness, palpitations, diaphoresis, orthostasis, seizure, extrapyramidal side effects, anti-cholinergic side effects, QT prolongation, suicidality

Pharmacologic Management

Treatment of pain associated with TMD can be non-pharmacologic and pharmacologic (Table 15.2).

Interventional and Surgical Management

Trigger point and Botox A injections may be beneficial for patients with dysfunction in the muscles of mastication. Surgical consult should be considered to evaluate if TMJ arthrocentesis or replacement is appropriate [3].

Functional Abdominal Pain and Irritable Bowel Syndrome

Functional abdominal pain (FAP) and Irritable Bowel Syndrome (IBS) both include symptoms of abdominal pain without an organic cause or features of somatization disorder. The key differences that distinguish FAP from IBS include continuous pain without association to eating or defecation. IBS is a multi-factorial process attributed to infection, altered gut motility and microbiology, stress and psychological comorbidities, visceral hypersensitivity, alterations in brain–gut connectivity and new evidence of altered peripheral immune function. The etiology of FAP involves a dysregulation between visceral input leading to peripheral hyperalgesia and eventually, alterations in central ascending and descending pain pathways [4].

Conservative Management

Initial treatments strategies should focus on gut motility and stress management by incorporating laxatives, fiber, diet modification, probiotics and daily exercise [4].

Table 15.3 Pharmacologic treatment options, mechanisms of action and associated side effects for FAP

Medication	Mechanism of action	Side effects
Tricyclic anti-depressants 1. Nortriptyline 2. Amitriptyline	− Increase serotonin and norepinephrine to augment descending pain pathways − Block sodium channels − NMDA antagonist	Drowsiness, dizziness, palpitations, diaphoresis, orthostasis, seizure, extrapyramidal side effects, anti-cholinergic side effects, QT prolongation, suicidality
SNRIs 1. Duloxetine 2. Milnacipran 3. Venlafaxine	Increase serotonin and norepinephrine to augment descending pain pathways	Nausea, headache, GI upset, decreased libido, blurred vision, weight changes, suicidality, serotonin syndrome, hepatotoxicity
Anticonvulsants 1. Gabapentin 2. Pregabalin	Block calcium channels	Dizziness, sedation, ataxia, peripheral edema, vision changes, weight gain, depression, Stevens–Johnson syndrome

Pharmacologic Management

Medications that can be used to treat pain associated with FAP or IBS are similar to other functional syndromes and chronic centralized pain syndrome treatments (Table 15.3).

Interstitial Cystitis

Interstitial cystitis (IC) is defined as chronic bladder pain frequently associated with increased urinary frequency and urgency.

Conservative Management

Patients should be educated on avoidance of bladder irritating substances such as caffeine, spicy and acidic foods. Symptom management also includes urinary alkalinization with baking soda or potassium citrate, increased water intake and bladder training. Application of ice or a heating pad in conjunction with pelvic floor physical therapy is also beneficial. Consider psychiatric consult to address associated anxiety and stress [5].

Pharmacologic Management

The pain associated with IC responds to pharmacologic therapy (Table 15.4).

Table 15.4 Pharmacologic treatment options, mechanisms of action and associated side effects for interstitial cystitis

Medication	Mechanism of action	Side effects
Tricyclic antidepressants 1. Nortriptyline 2. Amitriptyline	– Increase serotonin and norepinephrine to augment descending pain pathways – Block sodium channels – NMDA antagonist	Nausea, headache, GI upset, decreased libido, blurred vision, weight changes, suicidality, serotonin syndrome, hepatotoxicity
SNRIs 1. Duloxetine 2. Milnacipran 3. Venlafaxine	Increase serotonin and norepinephrine to augment descending pain pathways	Drowsiness, dizziness, palpitations, diaphoresis, orthostasis, seizure, extrapyramidal side effects, anti-cholinergic side effects, QT prolongation, suicidality
Histamine antagonists 1. Cimetidine 2. Hydroxyzine	Prevent histamine release by blocking mast cell degranulation	Headache, GI upset, dizziness, confusion, arrhythmias, seizure
Pentosan polysulfate	Believed to repair urothelium glycosaminoglycans	Rectal bleeding, alopecia, GI upset, rash, thrombocytopenia

Interventional and Surgical Management

For patients with refractory symptoms, consider urological consult for intravesicular dimethyl sulfoxide/heparin/lidocaine, cystoscopy with hydrodistension or intra-detrusor Botox A [5].

Chronic Pelvic Pain

Chronic pelvic pain is defined as a persistent, severe and distressing pelvic pain that has been present for 6 months. It can have a waxing and waning course or remain relatively constant but typically causes a change in quality of life. Patients frequently suffer from and should undergo treatment for a co-existing psychiatric disease such as anxiety or depression or a history of sexual abuse.

Pharmacologic Management

Chronic pelvic pain pharmacologic treatment can be effective for mild to moderate pain (Table 15.5).

Interventional Management

Depending on the location of the patient's pain consider a trial of caudal epidural, pudendal nerve block, or hypogastric plexus block.

Table 15.5 Pharmacologic treatment options, mechanisms of action and associated side effects for chronic pelvic pain

Medication class	Mechanism of action	Side effects
Acetaminophen	Unknown	Nausea, rash, hepatotoxicity
Non-steroidal anti-inflammatories	Inhibits cyclooxygenase, decreases prostaglandin and thromboxane	GI upset, GI bleeding, ash, hypertension, MI, nephrotoxicity, thrombocytopenia, Stevens–Johnson syndrome
Tricyclic antidepressants 1. Nortriptyline 2. Amitriptyline	– Increase serotonin and norepinephrine to augment descending pain pathways – Block sodium channels – NMDA antagonist	Drowsiness, dizziness, palpitations, diaphoresis, orthostasis, seizure, extrapyramidal side effects, anti-cholinergic side effects, QT prolongation, suicidality
Anticonvulsants 1. Gabapentin 2. Pregabalin	Block calcium channels	Dizziness, sedation, ataxia, peripheral edema, vision changes, weight gain, depression, Stevens–Johnson syndrome

References

1. Claux DJ. Fibromyalgia. JAMA. 2014;311(15):1547–55.
2. Nijs J, et al. Treatment of central sensitization in patients with 'unexplained' chronic pain: what options do we have? Expert Opin Pharmacother. 2011;12(7):1087–98.
3. Furquin BD, Flamengui L, Conti P. TMD and chronic pain: a current review. Dent Press J Orthod. 2015;20(1):127–33.
4. Farmer A, Aziz Q. Mechanisms and management of functional abdominal pain. J R Soc Med. 2014;107(9):347–54.
5. Colaco M, Evans R. Current guidelines in the management of interstitial cystitis. Transl Androl Urol. 2015;4(6):677–83.

Case 6: Sickle Cell Disease

C. Terrell Cummings

Key Points
- Understanding the recurrent nature of acute sickle cell crises aids in developing a streamlined care plan.
- Recognition of historically heavy reliance on opioids to treat acute sickle cell crisis pain and the potential for the development of tolerance and dependence among patients.
- Understanding the high incidence of conversion towards chronic pain in sickle cell disease.
- Recognition of the impact of co-morbid psychological disease and societal factors in sickle cell disease.

Background

Sickle Cell Disease (SCD) is a genetically inherited disorder that causes an abnormality in the conformational shape and function of red blood cells. This mutation in red cell shape manifests clinically as a constellation of symptoms related to ischemic changes due to clumping of red blood cells within patient vasculature. Ischemic changes can manifest within any end organ system, and can lead to a constellation of long-term disabling symptoms and a reduction in functionality [1]. The disease predominately affects African Americans within the USA and can also be traced to people with Mediterranean, Indian and Sub-Saharan African ancestry [1].

C. T. Cummings (✉)
Momentum Spine and Joint, Arlington, TX, USA

© Springer Nature Switzerland AG 2022
D. A. Edwards et al. (eds.), *Hospitalized Chronic Pain Patient*,
https://doi.org/10.1007/978-3-031-08376-1_16

Symptom Clinical Manifestations

Sickle Cell Disease is characterized by the recurrence of episodic "crises", which can affect any part of the body. Most commonly, the presenting symptom of a sickle cell crisis is pain. Patient can present with any number of symptoms related to ischemic changes to end organ systems. Painful manifestations include, but are not limited to, acute chest pain, myalgias, abdominal pain from splenic sequestration, priapism, dactylitis, headaches, skin necrosis, and flank pain from renal infarction. Other equally serious co-morbid complications include the potential for thromboembolic events, bone infarction, stroke, pneumonia, and acute hemolytic anemia, which can all lead to grave outcomes if not properly identified and aggressively treated. Frequent acute pain episodes are associated with a high mortality rate and requires prompt evaluation in the acute care setting [2].

Hospital treatment teams for patients in SCD crises usually include collaboration among internists, hematologists, a pain management service, and emergency room physicians. Currently, there are no gold standard laboratory studies, radiographic findings, or physical exam maneuvers that can confirm the presence of painful symptoms. Likewise, patients that have experienced repeated episodes of painful crises may routinely present without clinical manifestations of tachycardia, hypertension, diaphoresis, affective changes, or other objective clinical findings suggestive of typical acute pain processes.

Acute Care Presentation Triage

Identification of a treatable inciting event is important on acute patient presentation to a hospital setting. Ruling out potentially concomitant pathology such as acute infection, bone infarction, thromboembolic disease, dehydration, acidosis or acute hemolytic anemia is essential for patient management. Although outside of the scope of this text, identification of potentially fatal events such as acute chest syndrome, splenic infarction, and stroke must be carefully and aggressively triaged and managed upon presentation to an acute care setting [1].

Management of Acute Pain Crisis

Given the high frequency of recurrence of acute painful episodes, it is common practice for sickle cell patients to have an anticipatory pain management plan developed in conjunction with their primary hematologist to be executed in the home setting. It is estimated that up to 2/3 of pain crises are managed by patients at home under the direction of a previously devised health care plans. Patients are more likely to present to an ambulatory care center or hospital setting if their home plan fails to control their pain or if their symptoms are new or atypical from previous pain crises. Patients are also more likely to utilize the acute care setting during the transition from pediatric to adult care, in the age range of 18–22.

Formal recommendations for the care of acute pain crises for sickle cell patients was devised by expert panel and consensus guidelines in collaboration with the American Pain Society and the American Academy of Pain, published in JAMA in 2014 [1]. The primary treatment mainstay for acute pain episodes revolves around the delivery of multimodal analgesia management, with a traditional heavy dependence on the utilization of opioid analgesia. The use of multimodal analgesia is advocated as it allows for the targeting of the various neural receptors responsible for the transmission of pain signals. To note, there have been limited formal studies to objectively evaluate analgesia regimens employed for SCD patients with majority of recommendations formulated by consensus and expert panel guidelines.

Non-Opioid Analgesia Recommendations

NSAIDS along with Acetaminophen should be included in a multimodal analgesia regimen to reduce the inflammatory component of pain as is common with ischemic insults. For patients with significant muscle spasm, it is reasonable to include an antispasmodic. There is potential for ischemic changes at the neurovascular bundles which can predispose to neuropathic pain, thus the inclusion of an anticonvulsant medication, such as Gabapentin and Pregabalin, has proven to show additional benefit. Despite evidence that nearly 40% of SCD patients have a component of neuropathic pain at baseline, only ~5% are treated with an outpatient anticonvulsant.

Infusion therapy may be helpful for patients with refractory pain. Augmentation of inflammatory and neuropathic pain can be achieved with the adjunctive utilization of lidocaine as an infusion, with a retrospective study from 2015 demonstrating a >20% decreased in pain among patients receiving lidocaine infusions in over 50% of patients enrolled. Likewise, NMDA antagonism using sub-anesthetic doses of continuous ketamine infusion can be helpful, with recent evidence demonstrating reduction in pain and MME. Benefit is greater when used for young, male patients with longer duration of infusions. Magnesium infusions and topical lidocaine patches have failed to demonstrate an overall significant improvement in analgesia.

Neuraxial analgesia has been demonstrated as an effective adjunct in multiple case reports for SCD patients receiving continuous epidural analgesia during an acute crisis. This may be most helpful for patients with acute chest syndrome and compromised respiratory function, as well as for cases of abdominal pain and priapism, likely due to the vasodilatory effects of epidurally administered medications.

Role for Opioid Use for Acute Management of Pain

The use of opioids as a mainstay for the management of acute pain crises remains controversial but is universally accepted as apart of a first line therapy regimen. Patients should be provided with comprehensive and timely administration of medications to reduce pain while also minimizing unintended side effects of euphoria, sedation, and respiratory depression. It is recommended that parenteral opioid analgesia be a part of the patient treatment plan to facilitate early and rapid decline in pain severity due to maximum peak plasma levels and to better facilitate transition to oral analgesics [2].

The use of a PCA opioid has been widely used due to ease of medication administration and to improve patient satisfaction, despite concerns regarding the use of PCAs potentially prolonging hospitalization and increasing exposure to opioids, leading to tolerance. There remains controversy regarding the use of basal continuous opioid infusions vs. demand only infusions, as well as combinations with oral opioids. One study specifically assessing differences among prescribing practices saw a reduction in overall hospital stay (8.4 days vs. 10) for patients managed with demand only PCAs with a basal use of home long acting opioid formulation vs. continuous PCA infusion, and found no difference in hospital readmission rates in either 7 or 30 day follow up periods. Another RCT comparing high-dose demand bolus with low dose continuous PCA infusion versus low dose demand PCA bolus with a high dose basal rate provided weak evidence of quicker pain relief with the latter group over a 3-day time period [3].

Once patients have experienced a reduction of their pain crises and are ready for transition to an outpatient care setting, the use of oral opioids is preferred. Care should be carefully coordinated with patient's outpatient hematologist for medication maintenance and tapering to prevent potential long term sequalae of dependence and potential conversion to, or the enhancement of chronic pain.

It is to be expected that the majority of adult SCD patients develop tolerance to opioids due to frequent exposure during their lifetime due to sickle crises. Providers should be cognizant of this likelihood and tailor their initial and subsequent doses of analgesics accordingly. To note, there have not been any formal scientific studies to date comparing the analgesic properties of one opioid to another specifically for the use in acute pain crises in sickle cell. Long term, higher exposure to opioids has been documented to translate into more chronic pain states, with patients prescribed more than 90 MME/day reporting higher levels of daily chronic pain and lower levels of health-related quality of life scores. Goals of chronic pain management should entail reduction of baseline dosing during non-crises to minimize impact of tolerance on care during acute episodes.

Monitoring of cardiopulmonary status is important due to risk of respiratory depression with the use of opioids, regardless of prior patient exposure and tolerance [2]. Other potential side effects include risks for toxicity and seizures from the active metabolites, itching, dysphoria, and the potentiation of acute chest syndrome due to interactions with endothelial cell functionality and increased permeability [2]. Considerations regarding the administration of an opioid of choice should be also made based on metabolism, given a higher percentage of sickle cell patients who are ultra-metabolizers of codeine [2].

Conversion Towards Chronic Pain

Because of repeated episodes of painful vaso-occlusive attacks, it is common for patients to experience a clinical evolution of their pain: from intermittent crises to chronic daily widespread pain. It is believed that irreversible tissue damage leading to necrosis contributes along with a strong neuropathic component of pain contribute significantly to the conversion of acute pain into chronic daily pain. Studies have shown self-reports of adult patients with greater than 50% of days with chronic sickle cell related pain [1]. Chronic daily pain can be experienced in widespread locations to include the back, chest, extremities, non-healing ulcers, and bony infarctions; and frequently manifests in many patients by the time they enter early adulthood.

Chronic Opioid Therapy

Given a historic heavy reliance on opioids for treatment of SCD related pain, it is common for many patients to be maintained on a chronic opioid home regimen per their primary hematologist. Specific home treatment plans are aimed at reducing the frequency of acute pain episodes and to potentially self-treat mild to moderate episodes in the home. As previously mentioned, chronic opioid use may manifest as opioid tolerance and can lead to dependence among many patients battling this disease. Likewise, chronic use increases the incidence of central sensitization and opioid induced hyperalgesia. Central sensitization has demonstrable effects on reported pain severity, quality of life metrics, and can contribute to a cycle of stronger reliance on chronic opioid use and dependence. It is important to note that utilizing chronic daily opioids has limited evidence to support its practice and rather has been custom practice among sickle cell providers for decades. For this reason, there is a push for rigorous RCTs to definitively study the utility and necessity of this intervention to optimize prescription patterns.

Comorbid Psychological Disturbances

Providers must be aware of co-morbid psychological disturbances to include anxiety and depression. Similar to many other chronic disease states, there is evidence for a higher rate of mood disorders among patients with sickle cell anemia than in the general population, with many going without proper treatment and management. According to the PiSCES Study, co-morbid depression is more of an indicator for negative health outcomes in patients with SCD than genotypic mutation [4]. Studies have also demonstrated a greater daily reliance on both short and long-acting opioids for patients with negative affect, poor coping skills, and catastrophizing, which can further confound psychological disturbances. Many patients have self-reported home adjustments of their regimen to fit fluctuations in their daily affect; which is concerning due to increased risk for unintentional overdose because of psychological disturbances. It is for this reason that there is a push towards greater involvement of cognitive behavioral therapy (CBT) both during and in-between acute pain crises to help patients modulate their experience of pain and improve coping skills. Research has also demonstrated a benefit from patient involvement in peer support groups, skilled-based therapies (e.g., acupuncture, massage, hypnosis, biofeedback), and there is strong evidence to support integration of CBT to influence pain perception.

Treatment Challenges

Management of patients with sickle cell requires acknowledgement of the negative stigma associated with the disease. Due to frequent utilization of healthcare resources and historically high rates of prescriptions for opioid medications, patients oftentimes are labeled as "drug seekers". This commonly leads to delays in the administration of appropriate analgesia therapy and the undertreatment of pain crises. Understandably, due to the reinforcement of the provision of opioids with pain crises, many patients can indeed become opioid tolerant and potentially dependent with ongoing use with ever-escalating doses used for daily management. Likewise, patients are often labeled as high maintenance and difficult given their long-standing interaction with healthcare providers since childhood, where many were overprotected by vigilant family members and providers alike.

Patients oftentimes have a distrust of the medical community given perceived inconsistencies in the administration of care. There is well documented evidence of a disparity that exists in the provision of healthcare among African Americans and Caucasian Americans [4]. As this disease predominately affects African Americans, there is a heightened sense of distrust among patients and providers alike [2]. Patients often complain that their symptoms are minimized and disregarded given the oftentimes lack of objective clinical signs related to pain presentation, and as such, this frequently leads to a delay in the seeking of healthcare intervention in a pain crisis. There continues to be an ongoing push for increased cultural competency training for providers to improve care delivery for patients living with sickle cell disease [4].

References

1. Yawn BP, et al. Management of sickle cell disease: summary of the 2014 evidence-based report by expert panel members. JAMA. 2014;312(10):1033–48.
2. Telfer P, et al. Management of the acute painful crisis in sickle cell disease—a re-evaluation of the use of opioids in adult patients. Br J Haematol. 2014;166:157–64.
3. Dampier CD, et al. IMPROVE Trial: a randomized controlled trial of patient-controlled analgesia for sickle cell painful episodes: rationale, design challenges, initial experience, and recommendations for future studies. Clin Trials. 2013;10(2):319–31.
4. Smith W, et al. Understanding pain and improving management of sickle cell disease: the PiSCES study. J Natl Med Assoc. 2005;97(2):183–93.

Case 7: A Cancer Pain Crisis

17

April Zehm and Mihir M. Kamdar

Key Points
- For a cancer-related pain crisis, a rapid pain assessment should be conducted, including information about pain intensity and prior pain medication use (Fig. 17.1) [1, 2].
- Pain management should commence immediately, often before additional diagnostic studies are considered.
- Parenteral opioids are the mainstay of treatment for severe cancer-related pain. Opioid selection and dose depend on many factors, including hepatic and renal function and prior opioid use [3].
- Providers should not leave the patient and family until the crisis is controlled. Bedside priorities include rapid medication titration and monitoring of opioid response and side effects [4].
- Consider non-opioid co-analgesics early in the management plan for a pain crisis to enhance analgesia and reduce side effects.
- Once the patient is no longer in crisis, quickly orchestrate further testing as appropriate to formalize the diagnosis and tailor your management plan.

A. Zehm
Division of Geriatric and Palliative Medicine, Clinical Cancer Center, Medical College of Wisconsin, Milwaukee, WI, USA
e-mail: azehm@mcw.edu

M. M. Kamdar (✉)
Division of Palliative Care, Massachusetts General Hospital, Harvard University, Boston, MA, USA

Division of Anesthesia Pain Medicine, Massachusetts General Hospital, Harvard University, Boston, MA, USA
e-mail: mmkamdar@mgh.harvard.edu

© Springer Nature Switzerland AG 2022
D. A. Edwards et al. (eds.), *Hospitalized Chronic Pain Patient*,
https://doi.org/10.1007/978-3-031-08376-1_17

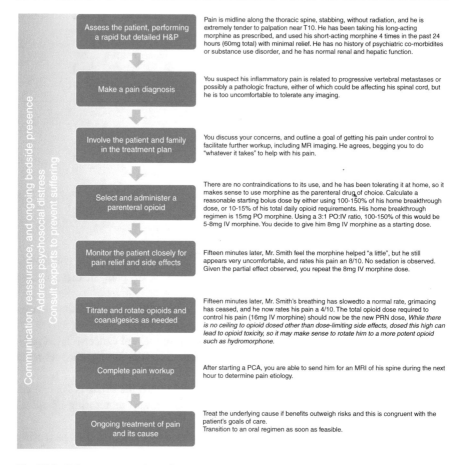

The flow diagram reads top to bottom with the following stages and explanatory notes:

Assess the patient, performing a rapid but detailed H&P — Pain is midline along the thoracic spine, stabbing, without radiation, and he is extremely tender to palpation near T10. He has been taking his long-acting morphine as prescribed, and used his short-acting morphine 4 times in the past 24 hours (60mg total) with minimal relief. He has no history of psychiatric co-morbidities or substance use disorder, and he has normal renal and hepatic function.

Make a pain diagnosis — You suspect his inflammatory pain is related to progressive vertebral metastases or possibly a pathologic fracture, either of which could be affecting his spinal cord, but he is too uncomfortable to tolerate any imaging.

Involve the patient and family in the treatment plan — You discuss your concerns, and outline a goal of getting his pain under control to facilitate further workup, including MR imaging. He agrees, begging you to do "whatever it takes" to help with his pain.

Select and administer a parenteral opioid — There are no contraindications to its use, and he has been tolerating it at home, so it makes sense to use morphine as the parenteral drug of choice. Calculate a reasonable starting bolus dose by either using 100-150% of his home breakthrough dose, or 10-15% of his total daily opioid requirements. His home breakthrough regimen is 15mg PO morphine. Using a 3:1 PO:IV ratio, 100-150% of this would be 5-8mg IV morphine. You decide to give him 8mg IV morphine as a starting dose.

Monitor the patient closely for pain relief and side effects — Fifteen minutes later, Mr. Smith feel the morphine helped "a little", but he still appears very uncomfortable, and rates his pain an 8/10. No sedation is observed. Given the partial effect observed, you repeat the 8mg IV morphine dose.

Titrate and rotate opioids and coanalgesics as needed — Fifteen minutes later, Mr. Smith's breathing has slowedto a normal rate, grimacing has ceased, and he now rates his pain a 4/10. The total opioid dose required to control his pain (16mg IV morphine) should now be the new PRN dose, *While there is no ceiling to opioid dosed other than dose-limiting side effects, dosed this high can lead to opioid toxicity, so it may make sense to rotate him to a more potent opioid such as hydromorphone.*

Complete pain workup — After starting a PCA, you are able to send him for an MRI of his spine during the next hour to determine pain etiology.

Ongoing treatment of pain and its cause — Treat the underlying cause if benefits outweigh risks and this is congruent with the patient's goals of care. Transition to an oral regimen as soon as feasible.

The vertical side labels read: Communication, reassurance, and ongoing bedside presence; Address psychosocial distress; Consult experts to prevent suffering.

Fig. 17.1 Pain treatment pathway in cancer

Treatments and Care Plan

Outcome

MRI confirms that Mr. Porter has new, multi-focal vertebral metastases of the thoracic spine from T8 to T11 as well as a pathologic compression fracture of T10, with no spinal cord involvement. You begin to discuss further management with him, including consultation of radiation oncology for possible palliative radiation, consideration of vertebroplasty or kyphoplasty, the addition of NSAIDs to his analgesic regimen, and transitioning to an oral opioid regimen as soon as feasible.

Multidisciplinary Approach and Considerations [5, 6]

- Analysis of pain presentation including the potential anatomical and physiological causes of pain based on comprehensive musculoskeletal and neurological exam as well as relevant studies (CT, MRI, PET, etc.).
- Treatment utilizing multiple classes of analgesic options can provide substantial analgesia with improved risk/side effect profile by addressing multiple different receptors along pain pathways. Synergistic actions of multiple classes of medications can provide superior relief than exaggerated doses of a single analgesic class. Options should consider, but are not limited to opioids, NSAIDs, steroids, anticonvulsants, SNRI/TCAs, NMDA antagonists, alpha agonists, local anesthetics, regional anesthesia, intrathecal drug administration, neuromodulation, and surgical treatment (DREZ, cordotomy, cingulotomy, etc.).
- Important to have discussion with patient, family, or surrogate regarding goals of care, as well as willingness to undergo various interventions for the purpose of pain reduction. Treatment plan should be personalized based on these goals.
- Expedient and often aggressive treatment is important in scenarios regarding cancer pain treatment due to acuteness of disease process and tumor burden. The likelihood or resolution of symptoms through normal course of time is less likely than with other medical conditions, with pain often increasing exponentially.
- Continue to reassess patient's response to treatment and analgesic needs, as these can change rapidly.
- Ensure adequate psychological support for both patient and family throughout the pain crisis and potentially thereafter. Important to involve an interdisciplinary team to assist with potential nonpharmacologic means of pain management and development of coping skills.

References

1. Foley K. Management of cancer pain. In: DeVita V, Hellman S, Rosenberg S, editors. Cancer principles and practice of oncology. 7th ed. Philadelphia: Lippincott Williams & Wilkins; 2005. p. 2615–49.
2. Harris D. Management of pain in advanced disease. Br Med Bull. 2014;110(1):117–28.
3. Carceni A, et al. Use of opioid analgesics in the treatment of cancer pain: evidence-based recommendations from the EAPC. Lancet Oncol. 2012;13:e58–68.
4. Moryl N, Coyle N, Foley K. Managing an acute pain crisis in a patient with advanced cancer: "this is as much of a crisis as a code". JAMA. 2008;299(12):1457–67.
5. Swarm R, et al. Adult cancer pain. J Natl Compr Canc Netw. 2010;8(9):1046–86.
6. World Health Organization. Cancer pain relief. Geneva: World Health Press; 1986.

Case 8: Spasticity and Pain

18

Peter V. Gikas and Meredith C. B. Adams

Key Points
- Spasticity is a neuromuscular condition relating to abnormal muscle tone commonly referred to as the property of velocity-dependent, increased resistance to passive stretch, thereby impairing movement.
- From a functional perspective, spasticity can be extremely debilitating, greatly impairing an individual's quality of life.
- Spasticity can significantly limit functional independence, as it can affect how patients ambulate, transfer, and perform basic activities of daily living.
- In the inpatient setting, spasticity can interfere with basic hygiene and nursing cares. It can promote muscle contractures, leading to an increased risk for the development of pressure sores.
- A spastic limb lends itself to the proliferation of heterotopic ossification, or bone formation at an abnormal anatomical site, usually in soft tissue [1].
- In contrast, spasticity can also paradoxically bestow functional benefit upon certain individuals, as its presence may also facilitate ambulation, standing, or even transfers.
- Spasticity is likewise intimately related to pain, as it can cause extreme discomfort in patients with intact sensation; it can promote fractures and even cause joint subluxations or dislocations.

Generally speaking, spasticity is a sensorimotor disorder caused by upper motor neuron (UMN) lesions. Spasticity is not to be confused with other movement disorders such as dystonia, rigidity, or myoclonus. The UMN syndrome is a collective

P. V. Gikas
Aurora Health Care, Milwaukee, WI, USA
e-mail: peter.gikas@aah.org

M. C. B. Adams (✉)
Department of Anesthesiology, Wake Forest Baptist Health, Winston-Salem, NC, USA
e-mail: meredith.adams@wakehealth.edu

© Springer Nature Switzerland AG 2022
D. A. Edwards et al. (eds.), *Hospitalized Chronic Pain Patient*,
https://doi.org/10.1007/978-3-031-08376-1_18

term which refers to an assortment of behaviors produced by lesions in the descending motor pathways of the brain or spinal cord proximal to the alpha motor neuron. Such lesions result in the loss of descending inhibition, promoting reflex arc hypersensitivity in the central nervous system.

Abnormal muscle tone in the form of spasticity is considered to be a manifestation of a positive sign (or abnormal behavior) in UMN disorders, as can be appreciated in an assortment of diverse pathologies. Other such positive signs include: athetosis, rigidity, dystonia, and the release of primitive reflexes (i.e. a positive Babinski response). Negative signs include weakness, paresis/paralysis, and fatigability (Table 18.1). Typical UMN syndromes in which spasticity regularly manifests, include spinal cord injury, cerebral palsy, multiple sclerosis, stroke, brain injury, and anoxic encephalopathy [2]. It is important to identify the presence of spasticity in this specific population set, as correct identification of this pathology can aid clinicians in the appropriate management of spasticity-mediated pain states, both acute and chronic.

Clinically, paresis and muscle weakness, collective negative features (or performance deficits) of UMN syndromes, usually accompany the positive sign of spasticity, making distinctions between paresis and spasticity difficult to ascertain. Nevertheless, concomitant muscle weakness and muscle over-activity coexist in UMN disorders, thereby affecting forces acting across joints shared in common by muscle groups, thus causing functional impairment and even pain. Spasticity can manifest itself in various ways, from very focal and localized digital dystonias to fulminant, generalized, spastic quadriparesis. Although clinically useful scales exist, such as the Modified Ashworth and Tardieu scales, spasticity has been historically difficult to quantify due to inter-user variability (Table 18.2).

Table 18.1 Signs of the upper motor neuron syndrome

Positive signs	Negative signs
– Spasticity	– Weakness/paresis
– Athetosis	– Paralysis
– Release of primitive reflexes	– Fatigability
– Rigidity	– Dexterity loss
– Dystonia	– Slowed movements
– Abnormal autonomic control	

Table 18.2 Modified Ashworth Scale

Passive Range of Motion (PROM) and Ashworth Scale (ASH):
Modified Ashworth Scale Key:
0: No increase in muscle tone
1: Slight increase in tone manifested by a "catch" followed by release
2: Mild increase in tone
3: Moderate increase in tone
4: Severe increase in tone
*: <10s clonus. **: >10s clonus

Treatments and Care Plan

Overall, treatment of spasticity aims to mitigate the positive symptoms of the UMN syndrome. Untreated spasticity can cause significant impairment in the performance of activities of daily living and mobility, often leading to irreparable muscle contractures, significant skin breakdown, increased caloric expenditure, neurogenic bowel and bladder, sleep disturbance, and even secondary depression. Additionally, noxious stimuli such as skin breakdown, deep vein thrombosis, urinary tract infections, and constipation often seen on the floor, can exacerbate spasticity (Table 18.3).

Over the past several decades, multimodal treatment strategies incorporating motor point blockade, chemoneurolysis, intrathecal baclofen (ITB) therapy, and botulinum toxin injections have been allied to traditional physical and occupational therapy regimens to optimize the capacity for maximal functional improvement in spastic patients. Treatment of spasticity begins in the acute inpatient setting, yet, often requires a lifetime to manage. Given that spasticity is a sensorimotor disorder, spasticity-mediated disturbances in both proprioception and sensation have been much more difficult to treat.

Managing pain due to spasticity is often quite challenging. Unfortunately, data with respect to prevalence, assessment, and treatment guidelines are largely lacking. Additionally, the basic science regarding physiologic pain mechanisms as they specifically relate to spasticity are not clearly delineated. In general, spasticity-mediated pain is thought to represent concomitant nociceptive and neuropathic pain mechanisms. With respect to the pathogenesis of nociceptive pain, multiple hypotheses exist range from unregulated muscle contraction in spastic muscles producing exaggerated oxygen consumption leading to tissue ischemia, that spasticity-mediated pain relates to an underlying mechanical and myofascial cause due to resultant weakness and generalized immobility implicit to UMN syndromes, or even that decreased inhibition of central neurons, and altered central processing may advance neuropathic pain processes in the context of spasticity.

With respect to treatment, the underlying pathology, a patient's cognitive status, time of onset, and the distribution of any abnormal muscle tone (focal vs. generalized), play an important role in devising an appropriate care plan. Therefore, a multimodal approach, including pharmacological and non-pharmacological interventions, is deemed most effective. Generally, spasticity should be treated conservatively, although surgical procedures can be considered in certain cases, namely:

Table 18.3 Factors that can aggravate spasticity	Pressure ulcers
	Ingrown toe nails
	Skin infections
	Constipation
	Urinary tract infections
	Deep vein thrombosis
	Improper positioning
	Ill-fitting orthotics

tendon lengthening or transfer procedures and even dorsal root rhizotomy. Typical initial treatment regimens include stretching/range of motion, splinting, physical modalities, oral medications, and local injections. Oral antispasmodic therapy continues to remain first-line (Table 18.4). A drug's side effect profile often limits titration to maximum therapeutic dosing.

Treatment of spasticity is most often attempted with the use of oral baclofen. In patients with severe spasticity, this can be problematic, given that only a fraction of the oral dose passes the blood–brain barrier, where target $GABA_B$ receptors lie, thus necessitating larger doses with a higher risk for unwanted side effects. Intrathecal delivery of baclofen, which requires surgical placement of an internal pump and catheter system, necessitates much less drug to achieve desired effects when compared to oral dosing. With respect to baclofen, recent data suggest that intrathecal baclofen may reduce spasticity-mediated pain better than oral therapy, especially diabetic neuropathic pain [3].

Over recent years, however, there have been a plethora of studies which have evaluated the effect of botulinum toxin (BoTX), a potent neurotoxin, on various pain states. Earlier reports hinted at the analgesic benefits of BoTX apart from its myorelaxant properties, with later studies demonstrated that botulinum toxin type A (BTX-A) involves attenuation of the release of neuro-transmitters themselves, including substance P, calcitonin gene–related peptide (CGRP), glutamate, and inhibition of vanilloid receptor activity [4, 5]. Additionally, BoTX has likewise been shown to ameliorate neurogenic inflammation, a process that results from sensitization of C-fiber nociceptors. According to a 2011 study by Aoki et al., BTX-A was determined to inhibit primary sensory fibers, leading to a reduction of peripheral sensitization, thereby reducing afferent signals to the dorsal horn and thus, indirectly moderating central sensitization, allodynia, and hyperalgesia [4]. Recent studies have demonstrated some evidence that botulinum toxin can be effective in treating post-herpetic neuralgia, postoperative or posttraumatic neuropathic pain, and even painful diabetic neuropathy [5].

Multidisciplinary Approach and Considerations

Spasticity-mediated pain can often be quite difficult to treat. The proper diagnosis of varying types of pain in patients suffering from spasticity, mainly nociceptive and neuropathic, determines the appropriate treatment strategy. A multidisciplinary approach involving coordinated efforts between primary care providers, physiatrists, pain medicine practitioners, physical and occupational therapists, and even orthopedic and neurosurgeons is needed to afford optimal results. Additional studies which further explore this complex pain syndrome are required.

Table 18.4 Common antispasmodics

Medication	Mechanism	Side effects	Uses	Cautions	Dose
Baclofen (Lioresal)	– Activation of pre-synaptic GABA$_B$ receptors	– Sedation – Drowsiness – Lower seizure threshold – Urinary retention	– Spasticity due to spinal cord injury, multiple sclerosis, brain injury	– Withdrawal can cause rebound spasticity, seizures, hallucinations – Renal clearance	– Start 5 mg qHS, BID, or TID – Can increase by 5 mg q3–5 days up to 80 mg/day (FDA max dose)
Diazepam (valium)	– Acts on GABA$_A$ – Facilitates membrane hyperpolarization	– Sedation – Decreased REM sleep – Memory impairment	– Spasticity due to SCI and MS	– Variable half-life – Hepatic metabolism – CNS depression	– Start 4 mg qHS or 2 mg BID – Fast onset
Dantrolene sodium (dantrium)	– Acts on striated muscle peripherally by blocking release of Ca^{2+} from sarcoplasmic reticulum – Fast twitch motor units more sensitive	– Liver toxicity in approximately 1% of patients w/risk of hepatonecrosis in females >30 years on doses >300 mg/day – Drowsiness – Weakness	– Spasticity of cerebral origin – Can also treat malignant hyperthermia, neuroleptic malignant syndrome, and hyperthermia	– Monitor LFTs periodically	– Start 25 mg BID – Total daily dose of 400 mg/day
Clonidine (Catapres)	– Alpha$_2$-adrenergic agonist – Transdermal patch and oral administration	– Hypotension – Syncope – Sedation – Dry mouth	– Spasticity due to SCI	– Withdrawal can result in hypertensive crisis – Impairs hypoglycemia-induced tachycardia	– Start patch at 0.1 mg/week up to 0.3 mg/week; change q 7 days – Start oral dose at 0.05 mg BID, up to 0.4 mg/day
Tizanidine (Zanaflex)	– Alpha$_2$-adrenergic agonist – Spinal and extra-spinal action – Enhances presynaptic inhibition of spinal reflexes	– Sedation – Hepatotoxicity – Hypotension – Bradycardia – Dry mouth	– Spasticity due to MS, SCI, or TBI – Less reports of treatment-related weakness	– Monitor LFTs – Short half-life requiring frequent dosing – Contraindicated with use of IV ciprofloxacin	– Start oral 2–4 mg/day qHS; max dose to 36 mg/day

References

1. Katz RT. Management of spasticity. In: Braddom RL, editor. Physical medicine and rehabilitation. Philadelphia: W.B. Saunders; 1996. p. 580–604.
2. McGuire JR. Epidemiology of spasticity in the adult and child. In: Brashear A, Elovic E, editors. Spasticity: diagnosis and management. Cham: Springer; 2011. p. 6.
3. McCormick ZL, Chu SK, Binler D, Neudorf D, Mathur SN, Lee J, Marciniak C. Intrathecal versus oral baclofen: a matched cohort study of spasticity, pain, sleep, fatigue, and quality of life. PM R. 2016;8(6):553–62.
4. Aoki KR, Francis J. Updates on the antinociceptive mechanism hypothesis of botulinum toxin A. Parkinsonism Relat Disord. 2011;17(Suppl 1):S28–33.
5. Wissel J, Müller J, Dressnandt J, Heinen F, Naumann M, Topka H, Poewe W. Management of spasticity associated pain with botulinum toxin A. J Pain Symptom Manag. 2000;20(1):44–9.

Jenna L. Walters

Pharmacologic Impact of Renal Impairment

Renal insufficiency and subsequently hemodialysis significantly alter the clearance and therapeutic levels of medications and their active metabolites eliminated by the kidneys. Varying degrees of renal impairment can increase the therapeutic levels of parent drugs and their active metabolites. Alternatively, patients with end stage renal disease may have a poor response to pharmacologic treatment due to drug elimination during hemodialysis. The degree of renal impairment, the accumulation of active metabolites and the elimination of active drug during hemodialysis are all considerations for the physician treating chronic pain in patients with co-existing chronic kidney disease.

Most non-opioid pharmacologic treatment options for chronic pain require some form of dosing alteration in patients with chronic kidney disease (Table 19.1). Most anticonvulsants have specific dosing guidelines based on creatinine clearance (CrCl). Gabapentin, pregabalin and topiramate are all primarily eliminated by renal excretion. Serotonin–norepinephrine reuptake inhibitors require dose reduction based on the degree of renal impairment and duloxetine is specifically not recommended in patients with severe kidney disease. Studies involving tricyclic antidepressants have shown accumulation of conjugated and unconjugated metabolites, but these metabolites are believed to be inactive [1]. Caution is still advised when administering these medications to patients with chronic kidney disease due to their side effect profile [1]. Muscle relaxants usually do not require significant dosing adjustment unless the patient suffers from severe renal impairment [2]. Both lidocaine and ketamine infusions should be used with caution in patients with severe renal dysfunction due to accumulation of metabolites and lack of published data, respectively [3, 4].

J. L. Walters (✉)
Midlands Orthopaedics and Neurosurgery, Columbia, SC, USA

© Springer Nature Switzerland AG 2022
D. A. Edwards et al. (eds.), *Hospitalized Chronic Pain Patient*,
https://doi.org/10.1007/978-3-031-08376-1_19

Table 19.1 Non-opioid pharmacologic treatment options, metabolism and recommended dosing changes in patients with renal and hepatic failure [1–4]

Medication	Metabolism	Dosing changes in renal failure	Dosing changes in hepatic failure
Anticonvulsants			
Gabapentin	Primarily eliminated in the urine as unchanged drug	Creatinine clearance ≥60 = 900–3600 mg/day >30–59 = 400–1400 mg/day >15–29 = 200–700 mg/day <15 = 100–300 mg/day *Re-dose after HD	No dosing changes recommended
Pregabalin	90% of drug eliminated unchanged in urine	Creatinine clearance ≥60 = no dosing adjustment 30–60 = reduce by 50% 15–30 = reduce by 75% <15 = reduce by 85–90% *Re-dose after HD	No dosing changes recommended
Topiramate	70% eliminated unchanged in urine	CrCl <70- decrease dose by 50% *50% reduction with HD (consider re-dosing)	Consider dose reduction in hepatic impairment
Lamotrigine	Metabolized primarily to inactive metabolite 2-N-glucuronide conjugate. 10% excreted in urine unchanged	Consider dose reduction in patients with severe renal impairment	Mild hepatic impairment- no dose reduction Moderate to severe hepatic impairment without ascites- reduce dose by 25% Severe hepatic impairment with ascites- reduce dose by 50%
Carbamazepine	Metabolized by CYP3A4 to carbamazepine 10,11-epoxide (CBZ-E). CBZ-E has eight-fold higher renal clearance the CBZ	Insufficient evidence to guide dosing in renal impairment *May cause renal dysfunction	Insufficient evidence to guide dosing in hepatic impairment *Rare cases of hepatic failure
Oxcarbazepine	Metabolized rapidly to 10-monohydroxy active metabolite (MHD) MHD excreted in urine either unchanged or as glucuronide metabolite	If CrCl <30 decrease dose by 50% No evidence to guide dosing in HD	Mild to moderate hepatic impairment revealed no pharmacokinetic changes of oxcarbazepine or MHD

Table 19.1 (continued)

Medication	Metabolism	Dosing changes in renal failure	Dosing changes in hepatic failure
Serotonin–norepinephrine reuptake inhibitors			
Duloxetine	Primarily metabolized by CYP1A2 and CYP2D6 to inactive metabolites. 70% of metabolites excreted in urine and 30% in feces	Not recommended if CrCl <30	**Not recommended** in severe hepatic dysfunction
Milnacipran	Primarily eliminated in the urine unchanged	Mild renal failure- no dosing changes Caution with moderate renal failure CrCl 5–29- reduce dose by 50% Not recommended in ESRD	No recommended dosing changes
Venlafaxine	Metabolized to active metabolite O-desmethylvenlafaxine. Parent drug and active metabolite excreted in the urine	Mild to moderate renal impairment— reduce dose by 25–50% ESRD—reduce dose by 50% and withhold until HD complete	Reduce dose by 50% in moderate hepatic impairment
Tricyclic antidepressants			
Nortriptyline	Primarily metabolized by CYP2D6 to less active hydroxy- metabolites. Metabolites primarily excreted in urine	Single study showed no significant difference in half-life or clearance in patients with CRF or patients on HD compared to normal controls Evidence exists for increased levels of both conjugated and unconjugated metabolites in patients with RF. **Use with caution**	**Use with caution** due to risk of accumulation of parent drug
Amitriptyline	Primarily metabolized CYP2C19 to nortriptyline and by CYP2D6 to less active hydroxyl-metabolites. Metabolites primarily excreted in urine	Evidence exists for increased levels of both conjugated and unconjugated metabolites in patients with renal failure. **Use with caution**	**Use with caution** due to risk of accumulation of parent drug caution

(continued)

Table 19.1 (continued)

Medication	Metabolism	Dosing changes in renal failure	Dosing changes in hepatic failure
Muscle relaxants			
Cyclobenzaprine	Metabolized by CYP3A4, CYP1A2 and CYP2D6 and metabolites excreted in the urine	No dose reduction required	Consider dose reduction in mild hepatic impairment **Not recommended** in mod to severe hepatic impairment
Tizanidine	Metabolized by CYP1A2 to inactive metabolites, which are primarily excreted in the urine	Caution if CrCl <25. Clearance reduced by 50%	Caution with any hepatic impairment. Monitor LFTs if used in patients with hepatic disease
Methocarbamol	Metabolized by dealkylation and hydroxylation Metabolites excreted in urine	Clearance reduced by 40% in study involving pts on HD	Clearance reduced by 70% in patients with cirrhosis
Local anesthetics			
Lidocaine	Rapidly metabolized to monoethylglycinexylidide and glycinexylidide: less potent but active metabolites. Metabolites excreted in urine	Use caution in patient with severe renal insufficiency not on HD	**Use with caution** in patients with hepatic impairment
NMDA antagonists			
Ketamine	Metabolized by liver to norketamine, which is approximately 20–30% as potent. Metabolites excreted via the kidneys	No data currently available. Case reports of safe administration in patients with renal impairment	No data currently available *May cause hepatotoxicity at high oral doses

Opioid pharmacologic treatment options also typically require dosing adjustments based on the degree of renal impairment (Table 19.2) [5, 6]. Alternatives to meperidine and morphine should be considered due to the risk of accumulation of active metabolites. Long-acting opioids should also be used with caution, especially in patients with severe chronic kidney disease [5, 6]. Buprenorphine is unique, in that is believed to relatively safe in patients with chronic kidney disease or those on hemodialysis.

Hepatic Disease

Hepatic impairment presents a unique challenge to the pain physician as almost every pharmacologic treatment option for chronic pain undergoes some form of hepatic metabolism. Specifically, the cytochrome P450 system are a group of hemoproteins that serve as a terminal oxidase in the electron transport chain. Additionally, many isoenzymes of the CYP450 system can be induced or inhibited by various drugs, which can impact the therapeutic levels of the medications used to treat

Table 19.2 Opioid pharmacologic treatment options, metabolism and recommended dosing changes in patients with renal and hepatic failure

Medications	Pharmacokinetics	Dosing changes in renal failure	Dosing changes in hepatic failure
Tramadol	Metabolized by CYP3A4 and CYP2B6 with one active metabolite O-desmethyltramadol (M1). 30% excreted unchanged in the urine and additional 60% as metabolites in the urine	Decreased excretion of Tramadol and active metabolite M1 CrCl <30, increase dosing interval to every 12 h and reduce max to 200 mg daily. No additional doses recommended with HD	Decreased metabolism of Tramadol and active metabolite M1 Cirrhotic patients, max dosage of 50 mg every 12 h
Meperidine	Metabolized by CYP3A4 and CYP2B6 to active metabolite normeperidine. Primarily renal excretion	Risk of accumulation of meperidine and normeperidine. Consider alternative	Risk of accumulation of meperidine and normeperidine. Consider alternative
Morphine	Hepatic conjugation to active metabolites Morphine-3-glucuronide (M3G) and Morphine-6-glucuronide (M6G). Primarily renal excretion	Risk of accumulation of M3G and M6G. Consider alternative	Consider dose reduction
Hydrocodone	Metabolized by multiple pathways including CYP3A4, CYP2D6, CYP2B6, and CYP2C19. Metabolized by CYP3A4 to primarily active metabolite norhydrocodone and by CYP2D6 to minor active metabolite hydromorphone. Elimination of hydrocodone and metabolites is primarily by the kidneys	Initiate at half the usual dose and monitor closely in patients with any renal impairment	Initiate at half the usual dose and monitor closely in patients with any hepatic impairment
Oxycodone	Metabolized by multiple pathways. Primarily metabolized by CYP3A4 to primary active metabolite noroxycodone and CYP2D6 to oxymorphone. Elimination of free oxycodone and metabolites is primarily by the kidneys	Initiate at half the usual dose and monitor closely in patients with any renal impairment	Initiate at half the usual dose and monitor closely in patients with any hepatic impairment

(continued)

Table 19.2 (continued)

Medications	Pharmacokinetics	Dosing changes in renal failure	Dosing changes in hepatic failure
Hydromorphone	Metabolized by glucuronidation in the liver with 95% metabolized to hydromorphone-3-glucuronide, which is excreted into the urine	Mod renal impairment (CrCl 40–60)- exposure to drug increased twofold Severe renal impairment (CrCl < 30)- exposure to drug increased threefold Reduce dose in moderate and severe renal impairment	Mod hepatic impairment- exposure to drug increased fourfold Severe hepatic impairment- not studied Reduce dose in moderate hepatic impairment
Methadone	Primarily metabolized by CYP3A4, CYP2B6, CYP2C19 to inactive metabolite 2-ethylidene-1,5-dimethyl-3,3-diphenylpyrrolidene (EDDP). Eliminated by extensive biotransformation, renal and fecal excretion. Extremely variable half-life (8–59 h)	Variable renal excretion of methadone and its metabolites. May be acceptable alternative in patients with renal impairment. Reduce dose and increase dosing interval	Consider dose reduction and increasing dosing interval
Fentanyl	Metabolized by CYP3A4 to norfentanyl and other inactive metabolites. Metabolites are primarily excreted in the urine	Avoid administration in patients with severe renal impairment. Start with half the dose in patients with mild and moderate renal impairment	Avoid in patients with severe hepatic impairment. Start with half the dose in patients with mild and moderate hepatic impairment
Buprenorphine	Metabolized by CYP3A4 to active metabolite norbuprenorphine and glucuronidation to inactive metabolites. Both active and inactive metabolites are excreted in the bile and urine	No differences found with administration of IV buprenorphine in normal patients compared to patients with renal impairment or on HD. Monitor closely due to risk of respiratory depression	No differences with IV administration in patients with mild or mod hepatic impairment Currently not recommended for patients with severe hepatic impairment. Proceed with caution in patients with moderate hepatic impairment

chronic pain. These interactions should always be considered when prescribing medications metabolized by the CYP450 system and dosing adjustments are recommended based on anticipated level of the parent drug and active metabolites.

Non-opioid pharmacologic treatments for chronic pain vary greatly in their degree of hepatic metabolism (Table 19.2). Several anticonvulsants used in the treatment of neuropathic pain undergo primarily renal excretion and are safe alternatives in patients with hepatic impairment. Serotonin-norepinephrine inhibitors and tricyclic antidepressants are typically safe but likely require dose adjustments, especially in severe hepatic dysfunction [1]. Most muscle relaxants should be used with extreme caution in patients with hepatic impairment due to the risk of sedation and respiratory depression [2]. Lidocaine and ketamine infusions should also be used with caution due to their metabolism and the risk of hepatoxicity reported with oral ketamine [3, 4].

Opioid pharmacologic options should also be used with caution and decreases in both dose and frequency of administration are recommended (Table 19.2). Meperidine specifically is not recommended in patients with hepatic impairment due to the risk of seizure with accumulation of its active metabolite normeperidine. Additionally, short acting opioids are likely a safer option as long acting formulations increase the risk of accumulation in chronic hepatic dysfunction.

References

1. Liberman JA, Cooper TB, Suckow RF, Steinberg H, Borenstein M, Brenner R, Kane JM. Tricyclic antidepressant and metabolite levels in chronic renal failure. Clin Pharmacol Ther. 1985;37(3):301–7.
2. Witenko C, Moorman-Li R, Motycka C, Duane K, Hincapie-Castillo J, Leonard P, Valaer C. Considerations for the appropriate use of skeletal muscle relaxants for the management of acute low back pain. Pharm Ther. 2014;39(6):427–35.
3. Capel MM, Jenkins R, Jefferson M, Thomas DM. Use of ketamine for ischemic pain in end-stage renal failure. J Pain Symptom Manage. 2008;35:232–4.
4. De Martin S, Orlando R, Bertoli M, Pegoraro P, Palatini P. Differential effect of chronic renal failure on the pharmacokinetics of lidocaine in patients receiving and not receiving hemodialysis. Clin Pharmacol Ther. 2006;80(6):597–606.
5. Pham PC, Khaing K, Sieveres TM, Pham PM, Miller JM, Pham SV, Pham PA, Pham PT. 2017 Update on pain management in patients with chronic kidney disease. Clin Kidney J. 2017;10(5):688–97.
6. Smith HS. Opioid metabolism. Mayo Clin Proc. 2009;84(7):613–24.

Case 10: Chronic Pain Patient After Spine Surgery

20

Christopher Howson and Meredith C. B. Adams

Key Points
- Preoperative opioid use can be associated with as much as a threefold increase in postoperative opioid requirements when compared to opioid naïve patients [1]
- While "pre-habilitation" has been shown to decrease post-operative hospital length of stay, there is mixed evidence regarding whether it has an effect on post-operative pain [2]
- Intraoperative ketamine can reduce perioperative opiate consumption in opiate-dependent patients; this has been specifically studied in patients with back pain undergoing back surgery.
- Multimodal analgesia using non-opioid medications (acetaminophen, NSAIDs, COX-2 inhibitors, anticonvulsants) can significantly reduce post-operative opioid requirements [3]
- When adjusting from oral opioid doses, most intravenous doses can be adjusted downward due to increased bioavailability [4]
- Use of partial-opioid antagonists/agonists or opioid antagonists should be approached cautiously in patients using chronic opioids as this may precipitate withdrawal symptoms

C. Howson
BayCare Clinic Pain and Rehab Medicine, Green Bay, WI, USA
e-mail: chowson@baycare.net

M. C. B. Adams (✉)
Department of Anesthesiology, Wake Forest Baptist Health, Winston-Salem, NC, USA
e-mail: meredith.adams@wakehealth.edu

© Springer Nature Switzerland AG 2022
D. A. Edwards et al. (eds.), *Hospitalized Chronic Pain Patient*,
https://doi.org/10.1007/978-3-031-08376-1_20

Review of Recent Literature

Over the past decade there has been a paradigm shift away from opioid-only treatment of postoperative pain; with attention instead turning towards multimodal management techniques. Even more recently, this emphasis on more comprehensive treatment modalities for perioperative pain has not only focused on what combinations of therapies are efficacious, but also the timing of such interventions. This has led to new research in the concepts of both pre-habilitation and preventative analgesia. Together these models take a proactive approach toward the treatment of perioperative pain by seeking to optimize the patient pre-operatively either through physical functionality training (pre-habilitation) or medication optimization (preventative analgesia).

Pre-habilitation is the process of improving physical functionality preoperatively to enable the individual to maintain a normal level of function during and after surgery. Despite the renewed interest in this subject, a recent systematic review published in 2015 by Cabilan et al. showed no significant postoperative benefits in function, quality of life or pain in patients who have had knee or hip arthroplasty [2]. This is in contrast to meta-analysis published in 2014 by Santa Mina et al. which showed that pre-habilitation may reduce length of stay and post-operative pain. Both of these study authors admit that further research in other surgical populations and higher methodological quality are needed to improve the external validity of these conclusions.

Preventative analgesia addresses the relationship between intraoperative tissue damage and an intensification of acute pain and long-term postoperative pain, now referred to as central sensitization. In a large meta-analysis, Ong et al. combined over 60 studies and then stratified the analgesic interventions based on outcome measures. The authors found the most robust analgesic effect for pre-emptive pain control was with epidural analgesia, followed by nonsteroidal anti-inflammatory drugs and local anesthetic wound infiltration. Importantly, increased use of pre-emptive opioids was not found to be efficacious. It should be noted that the duration and efficacy of a perioperative analgesic regimen has been found to be more important than any preoperative analgesic intervention alone [5].

Treatments and Care Plan

Despite heightened awareness by health care providers regarding the issue of pain management, data suggests that postoperative pain continues to be undermanaged with between 40 and 70% of patients describing moderate–severe pain after surgery. Achieving adequate pain control in patients already treated with chronic opioid therapy may be especially challenging because common strategies for alleviating postoperative pain may have diminished effectiveness. Nevertheless, early and aggressive management of pain is paramount because the intensity of acute postoperative pain has not only been associated with increased postoperative complications but also increased risk of chronic postsurgical pain. Patients already on chronic opioid therapy may represent a population that is particularly vulnerable for development of chronic post-surgical pain.

In an ideal situation, treatment of postsurgical pain should start with a preoperative discussion of expectations. Because the minimum daily opioid dose that significantly increases post-operative opioid requirements is not known, all patients should be informed about potential for aggravated pain and increased opioid requirements during their post-operative period. If, as is often the case, first discussion with the patient about postoperative pain occurs in the recovery room, the first step is often to establish the dosage of oral opioids that the patient takes at baseline. Patients should have received this opioid dose on the day of surgery, especially if large doses of long-acting opioids are involved, in order to avoid withdrawal and the need to "catch up" with the patient's opioid requirement. If the patient did not take their normal morning dosing of opioid, larger than expected opioid doses will be required initially in order to overcome the deficit and attain adequate pain control.

Assuming that the patient has already received their baseline opioid preoperatively and can tolerate oral dosing, postoperative orders should be placed which reflect a continuation of the baseline opioid dose, often in the form of extended release dosing, as well as short-acting medication for breakthrough pain. Total opioid dose per day, long acting plus short acting, should be started at approximately 25–50% more than the original dosage. Keep in mind that final opioid dosing may be up to 2–3 times that which would be required in an opioid naïve patient and that breakthrough doses will need to be titrated for each patient.

There are many instances in the post-operative period during which the patient may not be candidate for oral medication dosing because of the patient's physical condition, extent of the surgery, gastrointestinal function, and possible post-anesthetic sequelae such as nausea or vomiting. In such cases, conversion to either intravenous or intramuscular dosing is required. When switching routes of opioids, the goal is to achieve the optimal analgesia while avoiding the toxicity and side effects associated with overdosing as well as the inadequate pain control caused by under-dosing. When adjusting from oral opioid doses, keep in mind that most intravenous doses can be adjusted slightly downward due to increased bioavailability. In order to assist clinicians with this often confusing conversion, equianalgesic opioid conversion tables have been created (Table 20.1). Of note, the studies used to create

Table 20.1 Equianalgesic opioid dosing

Drug	Oral (mg)	Parenteral (mg)
Morphine	30	10
Hydrocodone	30	n/a
Hydromorphone	7.5	1.5
Oxycodone	20	10
Oxymorphone	10	1
Fentanyl	n/a	0.1
Codeine	200	100
Buprenorphine	0.4 (sublingual)	0.3
Meperidine	300	100
Tramadol	120	100

these tables generally utilized single doses and involved patients who had limited opioid exposure, thus may not extrapolate perfectly for patient managed with chronic opioid therapy. For this reason, it will remain necessary to assess for signs and symptoms of inadequate (unrelieved pain, withdrawal) or excessive (sedation, respiratory depression) throughout the perioperative period.

Because postoperative opioid requirements can vary immensely from patient-to-patient, it may be beneficial to employ an opioid-based PCA which will allow for the patient to dictate treatment of his/her breakthrough pain. Keep in mind that while use of short-acting opioids can be adequate for alleviating short lasting pain, their sole use in opioid-dependent patients may result in poorer results (i.e. opioid withdrawal symptoms can occur overnight if patient is asleep and does not activate opioid dosing for long periods). For this reason, a basal infusion of opioid may be indicated at doses comparable to their home dosing regimens. Titration of PCA dosing can often be initiated immediately after surgery in the recovery room, which has the benefit of closer nurse monitoring if changes to either the basal or breakthrough dosages is needed.

Multimodal Therapy

More recently, the use of adjuvant systemic analgesics (i.e. multimodal therapy) in the perioperative period have been shown to have opioid-sparing effects and as such may mitigate the side effects associated with high dose opioids. These medications can act on both peripheral and central sites to interfere with pain mechanisms that are different from the opioid system. Specifically, the addition of either non-steroidal anti-inflammatory, acetaminophen, or COX-2 inhibitor to opioid medication has been extensively studied in the postoperative period and shown to decrease both opioid requirements as well as decrease side effects. Perhaps more importantly, the combination of these medications is superior to any one component alone and their side effect profile is favorable, especially in patients without pre-existing renal or coagulation disorders. Of note acetaminophen has received special attention recently as there is now an intravenous form available in the United States.

Other adjuvant analgesic medications have also been evaluated for use in treating perioperative pain. In one study, a single dose of oral gabapentin (1200 mg) was able to significantly decrease postoperative morphine requirements as well as reduce movement-related pain [2]. Moreover, both gabapentin and pregabalin have been shown not only to decrease perioperative pain, but also to decrease the incidence of chronic pain more than 2 months after surgery; presumably by preventing the establishment of central sensitization as a response to the nociceptive stimulus of surgical incision.

In those patients who are particularly challenging either due to extremely high pre-operative opioid requirements or surgical pain refractory to more traditional medications, infusions of adjuvant medications may become an appropriate treatment option. Ketamine, an NMDA receptor antagonist is perhaps the most widely used infusion for treatment of intractable surgical pain and has been studied specifically on opiate dependent patients undergoing spine surgery. Loftus et al. showed that an infusion of ketamine intraoperatively decreased opioid consumption and pain intensity throughout the postoperative period without any significant side effects. While benefits on pain intensity may be more pronounced if the ketamine infusion is started intraoperatively, other studies have showed modest but still significant reduction in opioid requirements by using ketamine postoperatively, either as stand-alone infusion or as addition to PCA mixture. Dexmedetomidine, an alpha-2 adrenergic agonist, can be used as an infusion to reduce post-operative pain and opioid requirements. This may be especially useful in the treatment of patient taking chronic opioids because it can alleviate opioid withdrawal symptoms as well as pain.

In order to minimize side effects as well as polypharmacy, a regional anesthetic technique may also be an excellent adjunctive therapy option. Peripheral nerve blocks and epidural anesthesia have been well documented to reduce opioid-consumption as well as increase patient satisfaction in the postoperative period. Unfortunately, given the incision location for spinal surgery, traditional peripheral nerve blocks may be of little benefit. However, direct infiltration of local anesthetics into the surgical spine wound with a continuous infusion pump has also been shown to decrease post-operative pain scores, rescue medication requirements, and hospital length of stay. Of note, a single dose of local anesthetic placed intramuscularly by the surgeon intraoperatively during micro-discectomy did not have the same benefits.

References

1. Rapp SE, Ready LB, Nessly ML. Acute pain management in patients with prior opioid consumption: a case-controlled retrospective review. Pain. 1995;61(2):195–201.
2. Cabilan CJ, Hines S, Munday J. The effectiveness of prehabilitation or preoperative exercise for surgical patients: a systematic review protocol. JBI Database Syst Rev Implement Rep. 2015;13(1):146–87.
3. Clarke H, Bonin RP, Orser BA, et al. The prevention of chronic postsurgical pain using gabapentin and pregabalin: a combined systematic review and meta-analysis. Anesth Analg. 2012;115(2):428–42.
4. Mitra S, Sinatra RS. Perioperative management of acute pain in the opioid-dependent patient. Anesthesiology. 2004;101(1):212–27.
5. Vadivelu N, Mitra S, Schermer E, Kodumudi V, Kaye AD, Urman RD. Preventive analgesia for postoperative pain control: a broader concept. Local Reg Anesth. 2014;7:17–22.

Case 11: Angry Patient

21

Meredith C. B. Adams

Key Points
- Responsible individuals, when faced with the threat of illness can regress to childlike behaviors.
- In addition, with the abundance and accessibility of medical information nowadays, patients come armed with preconceived treatment ideas and expectations and a general distrust of the medical system when those expectations are not met [1].
- A patient with chronic low back pain may expect immediate relief when entering a hospital system and expect answers to why his condition has not been cured. Often times, the physician's decisions are also challenged.
- These adversarial encounters can generate negative feelings such as frustration, distrust, anxiety, guilt, and dislike within the physician [1].
- This can lead to reactionary conversations that further degrade the physician–patient relationship and escalate an already difficult encounter.

Evidence Based Approaches for Difficult Encounters

- Be aware of your own inner feelings and your reaction to these feelings [Level C]
- Try to stay non-judgmental and empathetic. Acknowledging their physical and emotional complaints and providing reassurance can improve trust. [Level C]
- Patient centered approach to interviewing or Motivational Interviewing. Mutual decision making. Recognize patient's goals. What are their needs, expectations? [Level B]
- Setting boundaries with your patient [Level C]

M. C. B. Adams (✉)
Department of Anesthesiology, Wake Forest Baptist Health, Winston-Salem, NC, USA
e-mail: meredith.adams@wakehealth.edu

© Springer Nature Switzerland AG 2022
D. A. Edwards et al. (eds.), *Hospitalized Chronic Pain Patient*,
https://doi.org/10.1007/978-3-031-08376-1_21

- Assess patient for underlying psychological disorders that can exacerbate pain [Level C]

A = consistent, good-quality patient-oriented evidence; B = inconsistent or limited-quality patient-oriented evidence; C = consensus, disease-oriented evidence, usual practice, expert opinion, or case series.

Treatments and Care Plan

Patient who suffer with chronic pain are often times reported to feel angry. Anger can further complicate pain management by disrupting the doctor–patient relationship as well as with other healthcare providers. In a study by Okifuji et al., assessing anger in patients suffering from chronic low back pain showed that 69% reported being angry at someone at the time of the study, with physicians being the second most common target of that anger [2].

The first step in resolving or preventing an escalation of a difficult encounter is to recognize which factors may be contributing, and thus highlight areas where effective communication can begin. There are three main groups (Table 21.1) the physician, the patient, and health care system factors that contribute to a difficult situation [3].

Approaching the Difficult Patient

You feel frustrated and annoyed by the patient and start to dread your visits with the patient.

Table 21.1 Physician, patient, and healthcare system factors contributing to difficult situations

Physician factors	Patient factors	Healthcare system factors
Sleep deprivation	Psychiatric disorders	Long wait times
Overworking	Drug seeking behavior	Negative interactions with
Compassion fatigue	Demanding/entitled	hospital staff
Poor communication skills	Angry/argumentative	Impersonal
Discomfort with diagnostic	Manipulative	Morning blood draws
uncertainty	Emotional, physical, or sexual	Uncomfortable beds
Negative biases	abuse	Lack of access to pain
Low level of experience	Anxiety/depression	centers
Inadequate training	Reluctance to take responsibility	Lack of accountability
Time pressure	for own health	
Abrasive and impatient	Belief systems that differ from	
personality	physician	
Insecurity	Financial constraints	
Anxiety/depression	Hypervigilance to body	
Personal health problems	sensations	
Discomfort with prescribing	Low literacy	
opioids		

The first step in managing a difficult patient is to recognize, acknowledge, and accept that these patient emotions are natural responses. The physician must then look inward and recognize how these negative emotions may affect how they are feeling. By taking a step back and controlling their own reactions, they can analyze the situation from a healthy distance, stay nonjudgmental, acknowledge the patient's feelings, and bring a caring attitude [1].

The patient feels the nursing staff is not on time with her medications and she is waiting around all day for answers. She is visibly frustrated.

De-escalating the patient's frustration is the first step to communicating effectively with patient to allow progress. Validating the patient's frustration by saying, "Thank you for being so patient. I can see you are in a lot pain. Let me see where the nurses are and I will let them know you are waiting for your medication." In many situations, acknowledging their frustration and reassurance is the critical first step. In addition, identifying environmental factors that may be contributing to the situation, such as "rude overnight staff," and working together with the patient to help alleviate these problems can prevent future difficult encounters. For example, you can tell the patient, "If you notice any issues again, please do not yell at my staff. Let me know so I can talk with my nurse manager to address this problem."

The patient questions every decision you make, is demanding stronger pain meds, and directs her own treatment.

In speaking to this patient, empathy is probably the most important tool in order to identify with and understand a patient's situation with chronic pain. Empathy can defuse a situation, build trust, and create an environment of mutual respect. A nonjudgmental attitude, active listening and patient centered interviewing can greatly improve the physician–patient relationship (Fig. 21.1) [4].

By listening to the patient, understanding the fears regarding their illness, the patient will be more likely trust the healthcare provider. Also clarifying the patient's expectations and having an honest discussion about finding common ground, working towards a cooperative decision-making process, and being realistic can further improve the doctor–patient relationship. This would also be a time to point out negative behaviors in a respectful and non-confrontational manner and explain how they may compromise the patient's care. Also, if their behavior is affecting your staff, this would be a good time to set boundaries. Threatening and overtly hostile behavior is separate from anger and frustration and should be handled according to local policy. At times unsafe behavior may require escalation and third party (security) involvement (Table 21.2).

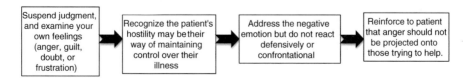

Fig. 21.1 Initial steps in addressing an angry or frustrated patient

Table 21.2 Communication strategies

Active listening and patient centered Interviewing	Understand the patient's priorities	"What are your most important issues to you right now."
	Let the patient talk without interruption	"Help me to understand why this upsets you so much."
	Clarify expectations	"What else can I do to help"
Validate emotions and empathize with the patient	Name and acknowledge the emotion	"I can see that you are angry and in pain"
		"You are right, you have been waiting for your medications. I will go check on it for you."

Adapted and modified from Cannarella et al. [5]

References

1. Strous RD, Ulman AM, Kotler M. The hateful patient revisited: relevance for 21st century medicine. Eur J Intern Med. 2006;17(6):387–93.
2. Okifuji A, Turk DC, Curran SL. Anger in chronic pain: investigations of anger targets and intensity. J Psychosom Res. 1999;47(1):1–12.
3. Haas LJ, Leiser JP, Magill MK, Sanyer ON. Management of the difficult patient. Am Fam Physician. 2005;72:2063–8.
4. Gorney M. The role of communication in the physician's office. Clin Plast Surg. 1999;26:133–41.
5. Cannarella Lorenzetti R, Jacques CH, Donovan C, Cottrell S, Buck J. Managing difficult encounters: understanding physician, patient, and situational factors. Am Fam Physician. 2013;87(6):419–25.

Case 12: Intrathecal Pain Pump

22

Christopher M. Sobey

Key Points
- Knowledge of potential causes of intrathecal pump complications is important when managing patients with these devices, requiring extra planning to avoid serious consequences to patients.
- Contact consultants early when encountering these devices to assist with management, including the managing provider and device company representatives.
- Device alarms need to be taken very seriously and with prompt determination of cause.

Background

Intrathecal drug delivery involves programmable implanted infusion systems (drug delivery devices, DDD; also known as targeted drug delivery) that deliver various pain medications into the intrathecal fluid surrounding the spinal cord, directly targeting pain receptors on the spinal cord. This allows direct action of pain medications in the central nervous system, reduction of total dose of medication needed, and potential for reduced systemic side effects of medications. There are multiple disease indications for infusion, ranging from diffuse widespread pain complaints to localized pain that is unresponsive to conventional treatment options [1].

Currently, there are two device companies who produce intrathecal infusion pumps.

Medtronic
- SynchroMed Pump I and II
- Accounts for the majority of patients with intrathecal DDD

C. M. Sobey (✉)
Department of Anesthesiology, Vanderbilt University Medical Center, Nashville, TN, USA
e-mail: christopher.m.sobey@vumc.org

© Springer Nature Switzerland AG 2022
D. A. Edwards et al. (eds.), *Hospitalized Chronic Pain Patient*,
https://doi.org/10.1007/978-3-031-08376-1_22

- Contact Number: (800) 328-0810
- www.professional.medtronic.com/pt/neuro/idd/prod

Flowonix
- Prometra Pump
- Patients should be wearing a medical alert bracelet
- Contact Number: (855) 356-9665)
- www.flowonix.com

Each of these devices provides sustained basal infusions with or without available bolus function [2, 3]. Patients with these devices implanted should have a Patient ID card that provides details. Moreover, patients with Prometra Pump from Flowonix should be wearing medical alert bracelets, which relate to MRI management. Once determined that a patient has a pump in place, consultation of the Pain Medicine team, Neurosurgery, or device representative to interrogate the device with a programmer is warranted (Table 22.1). This will provide further information including infusion contents, concentration, daily dose, amount remaining, and low reservoir alarm date. There are very important differences in the management of the devices, as well as potential system- and procedure-related complications that are important to understand.

FDA approved medications for intrathecal infusions include morphine, baclofen, and ziconotide, however, multiple medications are used as off-label treatment, either as monotherapy or in combination (Table 22.2). These off-label medications include, but are not limited to hydromorphone, fentanyl, sufentanil, bupivacaine, and clonidine. Determination of intrathecal infusion contents is vital to understanding management goals and risks associated with overdose or withdrawal.

Table 22.1 Management of an IT pump inpatient

1. Consult the pain medicine service/neurosurgical service/device company representative
2. Interrogate the pump to obtain:
   - infusion contents and concentrations
   - daily dose of medications
   - remaining volume
   - low reservoir alarm date

Table 22.2 FDA approved and off-label medications used in intrathecal infusions

FDA approved medications	Medications used off label
• Morphine	• Hydromorphone
• Baclofen	• Fentanyl
• Ziconotide	• Sufentanil
	• Bupivacaine
	• Clonidine

MRI Compatibility

Medtronic SynchroMed I and II pumps are MRI conditional. When the device comes into close proximity of the MRI magnet, the motor should automatically stall. The MRI can proceed as scheduled. After exiting the MRI environment, the pump needs to be interrogated to determine that the device stalled as expected, and then subsequently can be reprogrammed if necessary. If an interrogator is not immediately present, the patient can try to administer a bolus dose (if this function is enabled) to determine if the pump has resumed. If the pump is purposely stopped (rather than allowed to stall) and not restarted within 48 h, internal damage to the pump tubing can occur and replacement of device may be required. This damage will not occur if the infusion is instead programmed to the minimum rate setting, which is 0.006 mL/day for SynchroMed II pumps.

Flowonix Prometra I and II pumps are also MRI conditional, however prior to entering the MRI environment, the pump *has to be emptied* of the infusion solution, as the magnetic field can cause the pump valve to open, resulting in immediate discharge and drug overdose. The medication should be refilled and the device reprogrammed after leaving the MRI environment.

Alarming Pump

Both device manufactures have two distinct alarms for critical and non-critical alerts (Table 22.3).

In SynchroMed pumps by Medtronic, non-critical alarms are signified by 1 beep in variable increments from 1 to 6 h, whereas critical alarms are 2 beeps that can be set in variable increments from 10 min to 2 h.

In Prometra pumps by Flowonix, non-critical alarms are alerted by sounding two short (¼ s) beeps every 30 min, and critical alarms sound 3 long (1/2 s) beeps every 30 min.

When alarming, all pumps need to be interrogated and managed based on the alert. If a patient is discharged after management of an active alarm event, the patient should be closely monitored for under-dose or withdrawal symptoms.

Intrathecal Infusion Considerations

Patients with IT infusion devices have other special considerations. If patients undergo surgical intervention, the device should be interrogated before and after the procedure. Generally, it is suggested to maintain the basal infusion rate during surgery, keeping in mind the infusion of IT medication can contribute to increased sedation or cognitive effects from anesthesia. Short wave diathermy such as RF or electrocautery, should not be used within 30 cm of the pump or catheter [1].

Table 22.3 Managing complications

Issue	Possible causes	Management
Respiratory depression +/− CNS depression	Opioid overdose	Respiratory resuscitation +/− naloxone; determine cause (programming error, pocket fill, pump malfunction)
Drowsiness, lightheadedness, dizziness, somnolence, respiratory depression, seizures, hypotonia	Baclofen overdose	Maintain airway; empty pump reservoir consider withdrawing 30–40 cc CSF by lumbar puncture
Pruritis without rash, hypotension, paresthesias, fever, fever, altered mental state rebound spasticity, rhabdomyolysis	Baclofen under-dose/ withdrawal	Contact physician managing therapy; consider high dose oral or enteral baclofen vs restarting intrathecal baclofen vs. IV benzodiazepine infusion
Critical alarm	– Empty reservoir – End of service – Motor stall – Tube set interval – Critical pump memory – Error – Pump reset	Interrogate pump to determine cause of alarm; treat accordingly
Non-critical alarm	– Low reservoir – Elective replacement indicator – Non-critical pump memory error	Interrogate pump to determine cause of alarm; treat accordingly
Causes of overdose	– Pocket fill (subcutaneous bolus administration) – Inadvertent injection into Catheter Access Port – Pump malfunction – Programming error – Incorrect drug or concentration	
Causes of under-dose	– Catheter tear, break, or dislodgement – Catheter occlusion – Pump motor stall – Programming error – Battery depletion – Incorrect drug or concentration – Low reservoir volume – Missed refill appointment – Granuloma at end of catheter	

Dispersion pads should not be placed near the device, and the device should not be in between the surgical site and the dispersion pad. Knowledge of catheter location is important in surgical planning, in order to avoid inadvertent catheter damage during exposure.

Case Scenario

In the scenario with a patient with an intrathecal pain pump who presents with acute pain exacerbation such as trauma or pain crisis, after interrogating the device to ensure proper function, generally it is recommended to maintain the current settings and treat the acute exacerbation with IV or PO medications. If the pump dose needs to be changed in order to control the patient's pain appropriately, it is vital to communicate any alterations with the provider managing the device, as it would have implications for monitoring and alteration of refill date.

References

1. Deer TR, Pope JE, Hayek SM, et al. The Polyanalgesic Consensus Conference (PACC): Recommendations on intrathecal drug infusion systems best practices and guidelines. Neuromodulation. 2017;20:96–132.
2. Flowonix Medical Inc. Prometra II Programmable Pump. Budd Lake: Flowonix Medical; 2015.
3. Medtronic, Inc. SynchroMed II infusion system programming reference guide. Dublin: Medtronic; 2012.

Case 13: Spinal Cord Stimulation

23

Melissa McKittrick, Atish Patel, and Christopher M. Sobey

Key Points
- An understanding of SCS device function and components is essential for safe, effective management of patients with problems relating to and independent of SCS.
- The most common complication of SCS is lead migration, which usually leads to loss of paresthesia coverage (and thus recurrence of chronic pain).
- Epidural hematoma is a rare but serious complication of SCS, as it is associated with significant morbidity/mortality and requires emergent surgical evacuation.

Background

The concept of using electricity to treat pain dates back several millennia to the ancient Greeks, who applied live torpedo fish to the skin to treat headaches and joint pain [1]. Spinal cord and peripheral nerve stimulation techniques have been practiced since 1967, and improved safety and efficacy have made them increasingly popular, especially in the treatment of chronic pain with neuropathic components. Indications for SCS include failed back surgery syndrome with radicular pain, complex regional pain syndrome, peripheral neuropathy, phantom limb pain, chronic angina pectoris refractory to conventional management, and peripheral ischemic limb pain, however alternative indications continue to be investigated. Among other benefits, SCS implantation have been shown to significantly improve patient's health-related quality of life and treat pain in a cost-effective manner [2].

M. McKittrick (✉) · C. M. Sobey
Department of Anesthesiology, Vanderbilt University Medical Center, Nashville, TN, USA
e-mail: m.mckittrick@vumc.org; christopher.m.sobey@vumc.org

A. Patel
Department of Anesthesiology, Northwestern Medical Center, Chicago, IL, USA

© Springer Nature Switzerland AG 2022
D. A. Edwards et al. (eds.), *Hospitalized Chronic Pain Patient*,
https://doi.org/10.1007/978-3-031-08376-1_23

Despite decades of proven efficacy, the exact mechanism of SCS remains debated. Development and use was initially based on the *gate control theory* of pain, which proposed that non-painful stimuli inhibited 'gates' to painful stimulus, thus preventing pain sensation from traveling to the central nervous system (CNS). The assumption was that stimulating larger non-nociceptive afferent nerve fibers in the spinal cord inhibited the activation of smaller nociceptive projections in the dorsal column. Therefore, low-level electrical impulses (i.e. SCS) block nociceptive transmission, replacing a painful sensation with a paresthesia. This theory laid the groundwork for SCS-induced modulation, but recent investigations suggest that the mechanism(s) are more nuanced and may involve: inhibition of hyperexcitability of wide dynamic range cells in the dorsal horn of the spinal cord; increased activation of GABA-B, Muscarinic-4, and Adenosine-1 receptors; decreased glutamate and aspartate levels; and modulation of descending serotonergic and norepinephrine pathways. In ischemic pain, SCS appears to attenuate sympathetic hyper-activity leading to vasodilation. This mechanism lends itself to relief seen in angina pectoris with SCS, in addition to proposed mechanisms of cardiac conduction stabilization, adenosine release, and restoration of the oxygen supply-demand balance. Regardless of the mechanism(s), the impact is clear: SCS device implantation is increasingly popular, and as such it is almost certain that physicians will manage both hospitalized and ambulatory patients with these devices in place [1, 2].

To safely and appropriately manage patients with SCS devices, it is first important to understand device construct and function. The basic components of an SCS device include: electrode lead(s), an extension cable, an internal pulse generator (IPG), and a programming device. For trials, typically leads percutaneous (inserted via Tuohy needle) connected to an external IPG via an extension cable. Implanted SCS devices can involve either percutaneous leads or paddle (require open surgery) leads, with the leads connected directly to an implantable IPG, usually in the flank or buttocks. The IPG sends adjustable pulses to the leads that vary in amplitude, width, and frequency. Implantable IPGs come in essentially two forms: rechargeable and non-rechargeable. An external telemetry device can program the implanted SCS system via wireless communication, usually via low frequency RF signal.

Placement, programming, and management of an SCS device occurs as a collaboration between the patient, physician, and device representative(s). The pain history and location is of utmost importance, and this should be correlated with dermatome maps and current imaging. Following placement of temporary epidural leads, a multi-day SCS trial further confirms that formal SCS implantation should proceed. Patients should experience pain relief of adequate location and strength for the final operation to occur. After SCS device implantation, device representatives can help to identify what pulse qualities and mode(s) best cover patients' pain.

Risks

Despite their proven benefits, there are still significant adverse effects of SCS that are important to consider in the acute and chronic management of patients with SCS devices. A 2016 review article on SCS and peripheral nerve stimulation estimated a composite 30–40% incidence of complications. This article divided complications into those that were related to *hardware* (leads, extensions, IPG); *biologic* problems (infection, hematoma/seroma, hardware pain, dural puncture, nerve damage); and *programming* or therapy problems. They found that hardware-related problems were the most common, with the mean incidence (with a 95% confidence interval) including: lead migration 15.49% (CI 9.21–21.77), lead fracture or malfunction 6.37% (CI 2.63–10.10), and implant-related pain 6.15% (CI 0.97–11.33). Less common were biologic complications, with infection in 4.89% (CI 3.38–6.39). Therapy- or programming-related complications were often addressed via re-programming and rarely led to device failure. In the following paragraphs, we describe SCS device complications that are applicable to the management of hospitalized patients with chronic pain [3].

As stated above, *hardware-related* problems are more common and include lead migration and fracture, extension-related problems, and IPG-related problems (associated with battery depletion, flipping, or recharging) [3].

- **Lead migration** is the most common complication of SCS with reported migration rates from 2.7 to 27%. One article cited higher rates of lead displacement in the cervical spine, possibly due to higher mobility of this region. The usual consequence of lead migration is loss of paresthesia coverage; IPG reprogramming may recapture the correct sensory area, however reoperation is often necessary.
- Data for **lead fracture** is more difficult to separate, as it was often reported with lead malfunction or general hardware malfunction.
- **Extension-related** problems include disconnection or misconnection; these would manifest as inadequate paresthesia and/or pain coverage.
- When an IPG **battery is depleted**, this often necessitates replacement and thus repeat operation. Physicians in the hospital setting would most-likely see these patients presenting with worsening pain, or post-operatively after a replacement. It is considered a battery "failure" if replacement occurs before the expected date. Many studies don't include or report battery failure, so data is sparse on this complication.
- The IPG device is generally attached to soft tissue or subcutaneous fat, which presents the possibility of **battery "flipping"**, sliding, or otherwise moving. This can lead to device malfunction and/or be uncomfortable for patients.
- Some patients experience **rechargeable battery complications** such as unpleasant heat during recharging. Multiple short periods of charging (vs. one prolonged recharge) can alleviate this, but it may be bothersome enough for patients to have the SCS device explanted. Avoiding recharging for prolonged periods is not

recommended, as depletion without charging can lead to battery malfunction and require either a resource-intensive "reboot" or repeat operation for replacement. If a hospitalized patient experiences this problem, contact the device representative.

As stated above, *biological* complications are less common and include infection, hematoma or seroma, pain over hardware, dural puncture, serious nerve damage, and skin erosion [3].

- **Infection** is one of the most common SCS complications, with an incidence (mean 4.89%, range 2.5–10%) that exceeds the average surgical infection rate in the United States (2–5%). Device explantation is a "last resort" after less-invasive treatments (ex, antibiotics), but partial- or un-removed devices are associated with higher infection relapse and lower success rates. Furthermore, ongoing infection is dangerous: there are case reports of septic meningitis, aseptic meningitis, and paralysis secondary to abscess related to SCS devices. A review by Follet et al. reported that the most common organism was Staphylococcus (48%); the most common sites were IPG pocket (54%) and SCS leads (17%). Physicians caring for these patients should pay special attending to SCS device components during work-up for sepsis and/or infection
- Bleeding into the epidural space is rare but can occur when the space is accessed, leading to **epidural hematoma**; most case reports are after surgical paddle lead placement. Although rare, this complication is one of the most feared. One review article estimated the risk of hematoma development at 0.3% and the risk of resultant paralysis at 0.013%. Mortality after an epidural hematoma approaches 8%: 5.7% from the disease process and 2.9% from surgical complications. Epidural hematomas are surgical emergencies, as a delay in evacuation longer than 8–12 h from symptom onset portends poor neurologic outcomes. As such, physicians should have a high degree of suspicion when patients present with post-operative back pain and/or leg weakness, and emergent MRI with Neurosurgical consult is indicated [4].
- Other **serious neurological injury** can result from direct trauma during SCS device placement, such as during needle puncture or lead placement.
- **Pain over SCS hardware** has an incidence reported between 0.9 and 12%; of note, the study with the highest incidence used relatively large IPG devices.
- Dural puncture during lead positioning can lead to **post-dural puncture headaches**, with estimated 0–0.3% incidence. Symptoms include a positional headache, diplopia, tinnitus, neck pain, and photophobia. These symptoms hinder normal activities and thus confound assessment of SCS trial efficacy. Common treatments range from bed rest to a blood patch; as a last resort, surgical dural closure is an option.
- **Skin erosion** is another biological complication, with a reported incidence 0.2%.

Finally, *programming- or therapy-related complications* can cause loss of paresthesia or a new painful/unpleasant paresthesia. As mentioned above, these are usually addressed via outpatient re-programming and rarely led to device failure and/or explantation. However, they are symptoms that patients with SCS devices may describe during inpatient admissions, so it is important for all providers to be aware of them [3].

Considering the above complications, we will highlight below some possible scenarios that could necessitate SCS device troubleshooting in hospitalized patients.

Scenario 1: A patient with an SCS device presents to the ED with either abrupt recurrence of chronic pain, or new severe chest wall or abdominal pain. Consider lead migration which could cause loss of therapeutic paresthesia or new truncal stimulation. Management should include imaging to check lead placement, contacting the device representative (device may need to be reprogrammed or turned off), and excluding other emergencies (ex, pulmonary embolism leading to chest pain).

Scenario 2: An inpatient with an SCS device has declining mental status, and the primary team calls you to ask if the patient can have an MRI. Consider: the American Society for Testing and Materials classifies many SCS devices as "MRI conditional"—i.e. they "may or may not be safe...depending on the specific conditions." SCS device interactions with magnetic or radiofrequency fields can cause tissue tearing, device malfunction/failure, patient burns, and "noise" interfering with patient monitoring. Before the MRI, identify the type of SCS device, search for it on the manufacturer's website, contact the device representative, and consider putting the device in "MRI mode" if applicable. Discuss the safest MRI settings with the MRI technician or a Radiologist. During the MRI, establish direct communication and visual contact with the patient. Slowly introduce the patient to the magnetic field and ensure that the SCS device is not perpendicular to the MRI z-axis or close the MRI bore wall to avoid damage and minimize vibration. Post-MRI it is important to follow-up with the patient to ensure they experienced no adverse effects and that the SCS device is turned on and functioning appropriately [5].

Scenario Treatment Recommendations

For the chapter's introductory case scenario, the differential diagnosis would include epidural hematoma and epidural abscess, with hematoma being more likely given that that the patient is afebrile with unremarkable labs. As an epidural hematoma is a surgical emergency, you should order an emergent MRI to evaluate for hematoma. If managing an implantable SCS device, determine if the devices are conditional for spine MRI's or opt for a CT or CT myelogram. Neurosurgery should also be urgently involved so that they may evaluate the patient, review imaging, and prepare for emergent surgery, if necessary (best outcomes if within 8–12 h of symptom onset).

References

1. Compton AK, Shah B, Hayek SM. Spinal cord stimulation: a review. Curr Pain Headache Rep. 2012;16(1):35–42.
2. Jeon Y. Spinal cord stimulation in pain management: a review. Korean J Pain. 2012;25:143–50.
3. Eldabe S, et al. Complications of spinal cord stimulation and peripheral nerve stimulation techniques: a review of the literature. Pain Med. 2016;17:325–36.
4. Buvanendran A, Young A. Spinal epidural hematoma after spinal cord stimulator trial lead placement in a patient taking aspirin. Reg Anesth Pain Med. 2013;39(1):70–2.
5. De Andres J, Martinez-Sanjuan V, Fabregat-Cid G, Asensio-Samper JM, Sanchis-Lopez N, Villanueva-Perez V. MRI-compatible spinal cord stimulator device and related changes in patient safety and imaging artifacts. Pain Med. 2014;15(10):1815–9.

Case 14: Opioid Use Disorder

24

Rebecca Donald and David Marcovitz

Introduction

As of 2018, at least two million people in the United States over the age of 12 suffered from opioid use disorder (OUD) involving prescription opioids, heroin, or both [1, 2]. In this same year opioid overdoses accounted for 46,800 deaths, which is more deaths than were caused by motor vehicle accidents [2].

It is estimated that 2–6% of patients prescribed opioids for chronic pain relief will go on to develop some type of substance use disorder (SUD), while fewer than 20% of those with OUD specifically are receiving effective available treatment.

What Opioids Do to the Brain

When a person takes an opioid, the reward circuits in the brain are activated. Dopamine (DA) is the hormone in the brain that is released by neurons in the brainstem (ventral tegmental area or VTA) to signal the neurons in the striatum (nucleus accumbens) that something is rewarding or pleasurable. With repeated use of opioids, the brain circuits (mesocorticolimbic dopamine system) are changed so that anticipation of using an opioid, or even situations associated with using an opioid, trigger intense cravings. In addition, since the striatum helps the brain automate learned behaviors, patterns of use can become increasingly automatic with limited top-down control from frontal circuits. During opioid withdrawal there is intense anxiety and tension related to the release of stress hormones like norepinephrine and

R. Donald (✉)
Department of Anesthesiology, Vanderbilt University Medical Center, Nashville, TN, USA
e-mail: rebecca.donald@vumc.org

D. Marcovitz
Department of Psychiatry, Vanderbilt University Medical Center, Nashville, TN, USA
e-mail: david.marcovitz@vumc.org

© Springer Nature Switzerland AG 2022
D. A. Edwards et al. (eds.), *Hospitalized Chronic Pain Patient*,
https://doi.org/10.1007/978-3-031-08376-1_24

cortisol. Due to these effects of opioids on the brain, *impulsive* use of opioids (use that provides a positive effect) progresses to *compulsive* use (use to avoid withdrawal and stress). The neural circuitry of the brain has changed, and so the person is changed.

What Happens to People with an Addiction to Opioids

Compared to the person they were before using opioids, a person with OUD has reduced self-control (impulsive and compulsive), makes poor decisions (loss of executive function), has increased anxiety and stress, and has poor control over their emotions. Situations associated with using opioids and getting high become triggers and result in intense craving (conditioned reinforcement). Using opioids again becomes less effective at producing a high (a sign of tolerance) so the person may seek to use higher doses. Disruption of dopaminergic reward circuits means other stimuli are less pleasurable. In between use of opioids a person may go through withdrawal (a sign of dependence), and be stressed, depressed, or angry while preoccupied with using opioids again, at the expense of other choices (signs of addiction). Addiction can exist on a spectrum from mild to moderate to severe. Persons with severe addiction may have a difficult time being socially responsible, holding a job, or being a parent.

Vulnerability to OUD and Co-Occurring Psychiatric Disorders

It is now understood that although anyone can develop an OUD, there are predisposing factors including prior history of psychiatric disorders (especially trauma), prior SUD, or family history of psychiatric and SUD. Early onset of exposure to substances is also a risk factor. In addition, SUD frequently co-occurs with other psychiatric conditions. Of 20 million Americans with SUD, roughly eight million are also suffering from a mental illness. Substance use—including acute intoxication— is commonly linked with self-injurious behavior, with upwards of 40% of patients seeking addiction care endorsing prior history of suicide attempts. Though substance intoxication and withdrawal syndromes may resemble psychiatric disorders (e.g. dysphoria and anxiety from opioid withdrawal, or psychosis from acute stimulant intoxication), it is important that physicians ask about underlying disorders that may have been present prior to onset of SUD or during abstinent periods. Generalists and pain providers can initiate treatment and/or refer to psychiatric specialists.

The Best Way to Treat Opioid Addiction

The highest quality medical evidence supports routine inclusion of medications-for-addiction treatment (MAT) to promote the goals of recovery. The goals of recovery include: (1) decreased compulsive use of substances by controlling craving and withdrawal symptoms; and (2) improved executive control resulting in decreased risk-taking behavior, greater emotional control, and improved social functioning. Those who stabilize on MAT are more likely to meet these goals compared to those in other types of treatment alone or not in treatment. Medical treatment of addiction can be used for those explicitly seeking abstinence but also has a role to play in patients who are ambivalent about change. In both cases, medications reduce the chance of overdose death. For rescue, evidence supports the use of naloxone (Narcan) and its wide distribution for convenient use.

Treatment of OUD involves helping patients work toward abstinence from the misused opioid (prescribed, diverted, or illicit) followed by maintenance treatment to prevent relapse. Initial abstinence may occur by inpatient treatment in a hospital or approved facility, in the outpatient clinic setting, or during incarceration. Maintenance treatment may include either: (1) opioid agonist therapy with buprenorphine or methadone; (2) opioid antagonist therapy with IM naltrexone; or (3) psychosocial treatments alone without medication. As mentioned, treatment without medications can be successful for a limited number of individuals but should be considered in the context of how severe the OUD is, given the high rate of relapse and related mortality, especially with the proliferation of high-potency fentanyl. For example, incarcerated persons who undergo abstinence and then are subsequently released are at extremely high risk for overdose given the lack of tolerance to doses they were previously accustomed to.

The strongest medical evidence supports the use of methadone or buprenorphine formulations for maintenance therapy to retain patients in treatment, to control cravings, to reduce the risk of relapse, and to reduce the risk of overdose death. In the U.S., methadone treatment requires patients attend specially regulated Opioid Treatment Programs (OTPs), such that buprenorphine has emerged as an office-based alternative. Buprenorphine also has the advantage of a ceiling on respiratory depression when taken without other CNS depressants. Naltrexone is an opioid antagonist that does not cause euphoria or respiratory depression. It has not been shown to reduce all-cause mortality; however, it has been associated with a reduction in overdose events. Intramuscular (IM) naltrexone is an important alternative to opioid agonist therapy for some patients but can be difficult for many to initiate given it requires a greater period of opioid abstinence to initiate.

Patients who are enrolled in MAT are continually engaged with the healthcare community and thereby have improved health generally, due to health screening and treatment for other diseases. For these reasons, adherence to MAT has been correlated with lower overall healthcare costs among Medicaid patients.

Recovery from Opioid Addiction

The definition that is used for recovery determines how success is measured. For some, recovery is being abstinent from non-prescribed opioids, among other positive life changes. Opioid use disorder is a chronic disorder, meaning that, like in

Table 24.1 Memorizing the 11 criteria for opioid use disorder [5]

2–3 of the following = mild OUD 4–5 of the following = moderate OUD 6 or more of the following = severe OUD	Consider the "3 Cs" (compulsion, consequences, craving)
1. Overtaking opioids or using them longer than intended 2. Unsuccessful desire to cutback or control opioid use 3. A lot of time and effort is used to acquire, use, and recover from opioids 4. Opioid use in hazardous situations 5. Opioid use despite recognizing the problem	5 items related to problematic or **compulsive** opioid use
6. Opioid use is interfering with work, school, or home life duties 7. Opioid use is continued despite interfering with social and personal life 8. Opioid use causes the person to give up duties and social life activities	3 items showing the social impact of problematic opioid use (**consequences**)
9. Craving opioids 10. Signs of opioid tolerance 11. Signs of opioid withdrawal (dependence)	3 items showing the physiologic effects of prolonged use ("**craving**")

diabetes, long-term treatment may also be necessary. It is not well understood how long a person with OUD needs to be in treatment, or the timeframe for reversal of changes that have occurred in brain circuitry. However, promising research demonstrates that through MAT a person with OUD can regain executive function, indicating reactivation of healthy neuronal circuits.

The opioid epidemic over the past few decades has been met with increasing efforts to provide treatment for those who meet criteria for OUD (Table 24.1) with emphasis on inclusion of MAT. Though randomized studies thus far have not indicated that *requiring* behavioral treatments alongside MAT yields superior outcomes, 6–12 months remission rates in MAT treatment are only 50%, and so more research is needed to understand which specific patients require targeted behavioral interventions and stepped-care into more intensive treatments. Regardless, behavioral treatments should be offered to patients in MAT treatment whenever possible [3].

As indicated, providers must also pay close attention to management of co-occurring substance use disorder and co-occurring psychiatric and medical disorders in order to offer effective management.

Multispecialty engagement (e.g., Psychiatry, Pain Medicine, Palliative Care, Infectious Disease, etc.) and multidisciplinary engagement (e.g., including physicians, psychologists, nurses, social workers, and recovery coaches on the team) are both crucial when managing the complex co-morbid conditions commonly presenting in patients with SUDs [4].

Stigma: An Attribute, Behavior, or Condition That Is Socially Discrediting

Stereotypes and stigma often impact treatment [6]. Stigma is one reason only 10% of those with substance use disorder ask for treatment in a given year [7]. Stigma contributes to patient self-blame, and hopelessness. Stigma can also influence the medical care offered by clinicians who feel that treatment is ineffective or should be punitive, or who refuse to care for patients with SUD.

Some of the terms used to describe addiction unfortunately continue to promote stereotypes and stigmatize people with OUD and make it less likely they will enter treatment (Table 24.2).

When talking about other diseases, we say someone is a victim of their disease, suffers, endures, or is afflicted with the condition. A person dealing with cancer may be called (or call themselves) a fighter or a survivor.

Common potentially offensive terms used in the context of substance use disorders are labels like abuser, addict, junkie, or terms to describe labs test results or sobriety/relapse like clean or dirty.

Person-first language treats patients not as their illness (e.g. 'Mr. Gupta is a person with diabetes', instead of 'the diabetic in room 2'). Because language shapes thought and behavior, using non-stigmatizing language has a real impact on reducing the barriers to treatment and helping people feel comfortable to ask for treatment.

Opioid Withdrawal Symptoms

Opioid withdrawal symptoms can be very uncomfortable but generally are not life-threatening. However, the risk for fatal overdose during untreated withdrawal has led many to reconsider how we think about the urgency of opioid withdrawal.

Onset of opioid withdrawal symptoms following the last opioid exposure is variable and depends on the amount of drug used, duration of drug use, and half-life of the drug. In general, short-acting opioids cause more severe withdrawal symptoms than opioids with longer half-lives (Table 24.3).

Table 24.2 Person-first language to reduce stigma

Words/phrases to avoid (stigmatizing)	Person-first replacement (non-stigmatizing)
Addict/junkie	Person with a substance use disorder
Opioid addict/opioid abuser	Person with an opioid use disorder
Opioid abuse/drug habit	Opioid misuse/use disorder
Substance abuser/drug abuser	A person with substance use disorder
A baby born addicted to opioids	A baby born dependent to opioids
Urine was dirty	Urine drug screen was positive/negative for
Clean for 2 weeks	Abstinent for 2 weeks/in recovery
Detox	Medically supervised withdrawal

Table 24.3 Opioid withdrawal timeline of symptoms

Drug	Onset	Peak (h)	Duration (days)
Heroin	Within 12 h of last use	36–72	7–10
Fentanyl	Within 8–16 h of last use	36–72	5–8
Oxycodone/hydrocodone/morphine	Within 12 h of last use	24–48	3–5
Methadone/buprenorphine	Within 30 h of last use	72–96	>/= 14

Table 24.4 Medications to mitigate withdrawal symptoms

Symptom	Medication
Nausea	Ondansetron, metoclopramide; avoid promethazine as it potentiates opioids
Diarrhea	Loperamide
Anxiety, irritability, sweating	Clonidine (central alpha-2 adrenergic agonist that antagonizes the central sympathetic tone accompanying withdrawal); generally used at doses of 0.1–0.3 mg ever 6–8 h; maximum dose 1.2 mg daily
Insomnia	Diphenhydramine, trazodone
Pain	NSAIDS or acetaminophen for arthralgias

- **Early symptoms:** restlessness, irritability, anxiety, myalgia, abdominal cramping, watery eyes, lacrimation, rhinorrhea, diaphoresis, mydriasis, insomnia, yawning
- **Late symptoms:** tachycardia, hypertension, mydriasis, piloerection, anorexia, nausea, vomiting, diarrhea
- Patients may experience depression and cravings for opioids for a prolonged period [8]

The Clinical Opiate Withdrawal Scale (COWS) criteria are used to assess the severity of opioid withdrawal and to guide treatment with MAT [9] (Table 24.4). The criteria are:

1. pulse rate
2. sweating,
3. restlessness
4. pupil size
5. bone or joint aches
6. runny nose or tearing
7. GI upset
8. tremors
9. yawning
10. anxiety
11. gooseflesh skin

Important Points to Remember (Tables 24.5, 24.6 and 24.7)

- When used to treat OUD, methadone prescriptions are generally are not reported to prescription drug monitoring programs as they are dispensed to patients directly from federally regulated Opioid Treatment Programs (OTPs)
- Sublingual or buccal buprenorphine/naloxone (Suboxone) contains buprenorphine HCl and naloxone HCL dihydrate at a ratio of 4:1 buprenorphine: naloxone
  - The buprenorphine/naloxone combination was formulated to decrease IV misuse of the medication. There is minimal bioavailability of naloxone with sublingual or buccal administration, but it can precipitate withdrawal symptoms if injected by a current opioid user.
- Subutex is the sublingual formulation of buprenorphine that does not contain naloxone
  - Generally, Subutex is only prescribed to people who have a documented allergy to Suboxone and women who are pregnant.

Table 24.5 Evidence-based recommendations for treatment of opioid use disorder

Treatment for a person with OUD
1. **Medication**—includes buprenorphine, methadone, and IM naltrexone (MAT)
2. **Behavioral therapy**—includes psychotherapy (cognitive behavioral therapy, contingency management, 12-step facilitation) and recovery coaching.
3. **Lowering barriers to treatment access**—includes:
   a. Widespread screening, intervention, and referral to treatment (SBIRT)
   b. Emergency room and general hospital use of MAT
   c. Prison use of MAT
   d. Drug courts with specialty for women and families
   e. Law enforcement involvement
   f. Decreasing stigma
   g. Reducing delays in access to continuum of addiction care from outpatient to residential treatment
4. **Naloxone**—for overdose rescue, in hot spots, with EMS/LE, and prescribed
5. **Healthcare engagement for co-occurring medical and psychiatric disorder**—to improve MAT compliance, reduce recidivism, and improve general health
Treatment for those affected by another person with OUD
1. **Protocols for neonates born dependent on opioids** (NOWS)
2. **Behavioral health care access**—supportive significant other (SSO) therapy including Community Reinforcement and Family Training (CRAFT), Al-Anon and other community mutual help

Table 24.6 Annual cost of methadone, buprenorphine, naltrexone treatments in 2016 [10]

Program type	Components	Frequency	Per year
Methadone treatment	Medication and integrated psychology and support services (daily visits)	$126.00/week	$6552.00
Buprenorphine	Medication and twice-weekly visits for a stable patient	$115.00/week	$5980.00
Naltrexone	Drug administration and related services	$1176.50/month	$14,112.00

Table 24.7 Comparison of medications for OUD [11]

	Buprenorphine	Methadone	Naltrexone
Mechanism of action	Partial mu-receptor agonist with strong affinity for the opioid receptor. It will displace full mu agonists	Full mu-receptor agonist, although with weak affinity, so can be displaced by partial agonists and antagonists which can precipitate withdrawal	High-affinity mu-receptor antagonist Patients who use opioids while on naltrexone experience limited if any effect of the exogenous opioid
Phase of treatment	Medically supervised withdrawal, maintenance	Medically supervised withdrawal, maintenance	Following medically supervised withdrawal to prevent relapse to opioid misuse
Route of administration	Sublingual, buccal, subdermal implant, subcutaneous extended release injection	Oral	Oral, intra-muscular extended release
Metabolism	– Metabolized in liver mainly by CYP3A4; has less active metabolite, norbuprenorphine – Poor bioavailability when swallowed (< 5%) – Sublingual administration has bioavailability of around 30%		
Half-life		15–60 h	Depends on route of administration (PO vs. IV)
Usual dose	4–32 mg	80–100 mg	380 mg depot injection
Side effects	Headaches Nausea Constipation Xerostomia Respiratory rate can be slowed but has a plateau effect in adults		– Soreness at injection site – Possibly subacute withdrawal symptoms with first injection
Concerns	Risk of precipitated withdrawal	QT prolongation Respiratory depression	Risk of non-adherence, relapse, and subsequent overdose

Table 24.7 (continued)

	Buprenorphine	Methadone	Naltrexone
Advantages	Improved safety profile compared to methadone due to partial mu-receptor agonism • Suitable for patients with renal failure and those reliant on hemodialysis	May be effective for people who have not sufficiently benefitted from treatment with partial mu agonists or antagonists, in part because of intrinsic properties and in part because of program structure requiring daily attendance and behavioral therapy	– No misuse potential – No risk of diversion – Good option for people who do not want to be on any opioid
	When used as prescribed (buccal or sublingual administration) there is minimal bioavailability of the naloxone in buprenorphine/naloxone combinations		
Regulations and availability	Schedule III; requires waiver to prescribe outside of opioid treatment programs	Schedule II; only available at federally certified opioid treatment programs (OTPs) and acute inpatient hospital setting for OUD treatment	Not a scheduled medication; requires prescription

- Many patients will report an adverse reaction to Suboxone and request buprenorphine monotherapy. This may include a sensitivity to the taste of certain formulations. It should be noted that monotherapy has a higher street value given it is easier to misuse. Most patients can be educated about opportunities to try other formulations besides mono-product, and that naloxone is unlikely to be the cause of an adverse reaction given its limited bioavailability when taken sublingually. We caution against prescription of mono-product without a documented severe reaction to the combination product.
- Suboxone and Subutex are FDA approved only to treat OUD. These medications can provide an analgesic benefit to patients with OUD who also have chronic pain.
- Precipitated withdrawal can occur when a partial agonist, such as buprenorphine, is administered to a patient who is physically dependent on full mu agonists. Due to its high affinity for the mu receptor but its lower intrinsic activity at the mu opioid receptor, buprenorphine displaces any full agonist from the mu opioid receptor, but it activates the receptor to a lesser degree which results in the physiologic symptoms of opioid withdrawal. Precipitated withdrawal can also occur with administration of a mu receptor antagonist such as naloxone or naltrexone.

- Methadone, when used for OUD rather than for pain management, is typically dosed once daily. Sublingual or buccal buprenorphine should also be dosed once daily, though BID or TID dosing can be used for patients with co-occurring pain.

Acute Pain Management in Patients Taking Buprenorphine for MAT

Approaches vary and will depend on the patient's pathology and severity of pain [12].

Buprenorphine options for acute pain
- Continue same buprenorphine maintenance dose and optimize non-opioid analgesics
  - Anti-inflammatories
  - Muscle relaxants (methocarbamol, cyclobenzaprine, tizanidine, metaxalone)
  - Gabapentin/pregabalin for neuropathic pain
  - Consider TCAs/SNRIs
  - Sodium channel blocker: lidocaine infusion
  - NMDA receptor antagonists: ketamine infusion, memantine
  - Consider regional anesthesia
- Divide total daily buprenorphine dose into BID or TID dosing to improve pain control while treating opioid dependence
  - The analgesic duration of buprenorphine is only a few hours
- Temporarily increase buprenorphine dose and divide total daily buprenorphine dose into BID or TID dosing to improve pain control while treating opioid dependence
  - Plan for taper back to baseline dose after episode of acute pain has resolved
- Continue buprenorphine therapy and add full agonists to achieve greater levels of analgesia
  - May be minimally beneficial in patients taking over 16 mg of buprenorphine daily as > 95% of the mu receptors are saturated at this dose
  - If additional opioids are ultimately required, short-acting, high affinity full agonists (e.g. hydromorphone, fentanyl) may be used. These doses may be higher than normally expected, and thus appropriate monitoring must be available. When severe post-operative pain has resolved, taper and discontinuation of full agonist can proceed until the individual is ultimately only on the original dose of buprenorphine/naloxone
- Stop buprenorphine and initiate full opioid agonist therapy

Methadone
- Optimize multimodal therapy as above
- Divide total daily methadone dose into BID or TID dosing to improve pain control while treating opioid dependence

- The analgesic duration of methadone is 6–8 h.
- Consider increasing methadone dose temporarily. When severe post-operative pain has resolved, the dose of methadone can be decreased to the original dose and ultimately transitioned from TID dosing to BID dosing and finally to daily dosing.
- Consider keeping methadone dose at baseline and adding short acting opioids at regular intervals.

Naltrexone
- Patients on naltrexone will not responds to mu agonists in the typical fashion as the mu receptors will be blocked by naltrexone.
- Optimize multimodal analgesics (as above)
- Consider regional anesthesia
- For intractable pain not adequately controlled by other means, consider conscious sedation with benzodiazepines, ketamine, or general anesthesia.

Additional important points
- Because of stigma, there has been a significant risk that patients with OUD will have their acute pain under treated in the general hospital. These patients have increased tolerance to opioids and heightened sensitivity to pain and stress at baseline. For that reason, withholding appropriate opioid analgesia can be particularly difficult for them and can result in departures from the hospital against medical advice and other behavioral issues including hospital misuse of substances.
- When acute pathology is evident or uncertain in the first 24–72 h of admission, we do recommend that inpatient medical teams err on the side of treating acute pain assertively with opioid if indicated. This will also prevent neglect of acute withdrawal symptoms.
- Patients in sustained recovery on or off MAT may need coaching that brief use of prescribed opioids in the hospital is not tantamount to relapse. At the same time, providers should take a patient-centered approach and respect patient wishes if they wish to avoid opioids despite significant pain.

Treating the Pregnant Patient

Historically, methadone has been considered the first-line treatment for OUD in pregnant women. However, buprenorphine is well-tolerated and effective with potential benefits, including lower risk of overdose, fewer drug interactions, milder withdrawal symptoms with neonatal abstinence syndrome, and shorter hospital stay. Buprenorphine without naloxone has historically been recommended with pregnant women, though more recent data suggests that combination product is also safe for mother and fetus and safe during breast-feeding. Due to increases in circulating blood volume and increased metabolism, many women will require higher doses in the second and third trimester (and/or BID or TID dosing) with return to baseline dose after delivery. In the post-partum period, mothers can transition to their pre-pregnancy dose and formulation of buprenorphine. Methadone also reduces cravings and facilitates abstinence in pregnant women.

References

1. Mental Health Services Administration. National survey on drug use and health (NSDUH). Rockville: Mental Health Services Administration; 2014.
2. Han B, Volkow ND, Compton WM, McCance-Katz EF. Reported heroin use, use disorder, and injection among adults in the United States, 2002–2018. JAMA. 2020;323(6):568–71.
3. Carroll KM, Weiss RD. The role of behavioral interventions in buprenorphine maintenance treatment: a review. Am J Psychiatry. 2017;174(8):738–47.
4. Kelly TM, Daley DC. Integrated treatment of substance use and psychiatric disorders. Soc Work Public Health. 2013;28(3–4):388–406. https://doi.org/10.1080/19371918.2013.774673.
5. American Psychiatric Association. Diagnostic and statistical manual of mental disorders. 5th ed. Arlington: American Psychiatric Association; 2013.
6. Brezing C, Marcovitz D. Stigma and persons with substance use disorders. In: Stigma and prejudice. Cham: Humana Press; 2016. p. 113–32.
7. Kelly JF, Wakeman SE, Saitz R. Stop talking 'dirty': clinicians, language, and quality of care for the leading cause of preventable death in the United States. Am J Med. 2015;128(1):8–9.
8. Pergolizzi R. Opioid withdrawal symptoms, a consequence of chronic opioid use and opioid use disorder: current understanding and approaches to management. J Clin Pharm Ther. 2020;45(5):892–903. https://doi.org/10.1111/jcpt.13114.
9. Wesson DR, Ling W. The clinical opiate withdrawal scale (COWS). J Psychoactive Drugs. 2003;35:253–9.
10. Department of Defense (DoD). TRICARE; Mental health and substance use disorder treatment. Fed Regist. 2016;81(171):61067–98.
11. Substance Abuse and Mental Health Services Administration (US). Medications for opioid use disorder: for healthcare and addiction professionals, policymakers, patients, and families. (Treatment Improvement Protocol (TIP) Series, No. 63). Rockville: Substance Abuse and Mental Health Services Administration; 2018.
12. Kampman J. American Society of Addiction Medicine (ASAM) national practice guideline for the use of medications in the treatment of addiction involving opioid use. J Addict Med. 2015;9(5):358–67. https://doi.org/10.1097/adm.0000000000000166.

Case 15: Comorbid Psychological Condition

25

Gwynne Kirchen and Meredith C. B. Adams

Key Points

When considering a patient with comorbid psychological and chronic pain disease, it is important to assess the history and course of each complaint. Identify previous treatments utilized with their effect and the different specialists previously involved in the care of the patient (therapists, psychologists, psychiatrists, pain specialists, rehabilitation counselors). Assess for history of suicidal or homicidal ideation, history of and risk of opioid misuse (e.g., Opioid Risk Tool), substance abuse and medication combinations associated with increased morbidity and mortality including benzodiazepines and opioids. Anticipate the need for a multidisciplinary approach for both the acute and chronic care of the patient.

Literature Review

- Patients with chronic pain have high prevalence of comorbid psychiatric disorders, the most common of which is depression followed by anxiety. It is unclear whether the relationship between these diseases is concomitant or consequent of one another. It has been shown that pain and depression are both a risk factor for subsequent development of the other [1].
- Patients with comorbid pain and psychological disease are less likely to improve with standard chronic pain treatment, as identified by worse treatment outcomes and greater level of disability. Rehabilitation can be compromised if psychological illness isn't appropriately recognized or treated [2].

G. Kirchen
Medical College of Wisconsin, Milwaukee, WI, USA
e-mail: gkirchen@mcw.edu

M. C. B. Adams (✉)
Department of Anesthesiology, Wake Forest Baptist Health, Winston-Salem, NC, USA
e-mail: meredith.adams@wakehealth.edu

© Springer Nature Switzerland AG 2022
D. A. Edwards et al. (eds.), *Hospitalized Chronic Pain Patient*,
https://doi.org/10.1007/978-3-031-08376-1_25

- Despite high rates of psychiatric disorders, very few patients receive mental health treatment [3].
- Patients with high negative affect, defined as negative thoughts including depression, anxiety and pain catastrophizing, are shown to require higher opiate dosages with poorer analgesic response and higher risk of opiate misuse and cravings [4].

Case Scenario Care Plan

- After a thorough history and physical examination of the patient, a physician must address this patient's acute pain requirements. Continue and escalate opioids with a clear discussion with the patient of realistic pain expectations. The patient should understand the increased risk of opioid tolerance and hyperalgesia and how that will relate to his or her pain control. Outline and document a plan for tapering of opioids as the acute pain process resolves. Establish follow up with a practitioner comfortable with the tapering process.
- Utilize a multimodal approach to analgesia for the patient. Consider NSAIDS, acetaminophen, calcium channel antagonists (gabapentin, pregabalin), topical analgesics and regional anesthesia as appropriate for the patient's pain complaint and history.
- Consider initiation of neuromodulatory pharmacologic agents (Table 25.1) such as selective serotonin and norepinephrine reuptake inhibitors (SSNRIs), tricyclic antidepressants (TCAs) or selective serotonin reuptake inhibitors (SSRIs). Discuss with mental health expert to select a medication with appropriate

Table 25.1 Neuromodulatory pharmacologic agents

Class of medication	Example	Background	Side effects
SSNRIs	Duloxetine, Venlafaxine	Duloxetine was first antidepressant with FDA approval for pain indication	More benign side effect profile than TCAs
TCAs	Nortriptyline, Amitriptyline	Analgesic effect occurs more rapidly and at lower doses than mood effect	Side effects primarily related to anticholinergic effect. Most common antidepressant used in overdose, therefore may not be appropriate in patient with suicidal ideation
SSRIs	Fluoxetine	Less efficacy for pain complaint	More benign side effect profile than TCAs
Ca channel antagonist	Gabapentin, Pregabalin	Indicated for neuropathic pain. Requires titration to effective dose and dose adjustment for CKD	Most commonly sedation and dizziness that can be ameliorated by slower dose titration

balance of pain and mood effect without interaction with any currently pre-scribed medication. Educate patient about side effect profile, titration schedule and expected timeframe of efficacy [5].

- Organize multidisciplinary team including pain physician, psychiatrist, pain psychologist, physical therapist, social worker and surgeon as appropriate for patient's specific situation. Establish follow up with mental health care provider.

References

1. Korff MV, Crane P, Lane M, et al. Chronic spinal pain and physical–mental comorbidity in the United States: results from the national comorbidity survey replication. Pain. 2005;113(3):331–9.
2. Workman EA, Hubbard JR, Felker BL. Comorbid psychiatric disorders and predictors of pain management program success in patients with chronic pain. Prim Care Companion J Clin Psychiatry. 2002;04(04):137–40.
3. Barry DT, Cutter CJ, Beitel M, Kerns RD, Liong C, Schottenfeld RS. Psychiatric disorders among patients seeking treatment for co-occurring chronic pain and opioid use disorder. J Clin Psychiatry. 2016;77(10):13715.
4. Wasan AD, Michna E, Edwards RR, et al. Psychiatric comorbidity is associated prospectively with diminished opioid analgesia and increased opioid misuse in patients with chronic low back pain. Anesthesiology. 2015;123(4):861–72.
5. Smith HS, Argoff CE, McCleane G. Antidepressants as analgesics. In: Practical management of pain. 5th ed. Amsterdam: Elsevier; 2014. p. 530–42.

Case 16: Poor Prognosis in a Palliative Care Patient

26

Andrew Wooldridge and Myrick C. Shinall Jr

Key Points
- Effective treatment of patients with limited life expectancy requires attention to "total pain," the sum of their physical pain, other bothersome symptoms, and emotional distress.
- Patients with limited life expectancy may still be candidates for procedures or other treatment modalities, so appropriate specialist consultation is important.
- Multidisciplinary palliative care teams can include physicians, midlevel providers, social workers, psychologists, case managers, and chaplains. Each can have an important role to play in treating a patient's total pain.
- Patients with life expectancy of less than six months are eligible for hospice care, which can be provided at home or in a facility, and they should be offered the opportunity to decide whether hospice care is right for them.

Treatments and Care Plan

One of the most important considerations in addressing pain in the patient with a limited life expectancy is the concept of "total pain." This concept emphasizes that a patient's experience of pain depends not just on nociceptive stimuli, but also on the other types of psychological distress the patient simultaneously experiences. Patients with a life-limiting prognosis will often have other severe symptoms, such as dyspnea or nausea, that compound the experience of pain. Moreover, a poor prognosis generates psychological, social, and spiritual distress that complicates the management of pain.

A. Wooldridge
Department of Medicine, Division of Palliative Care, Vanderbilt University Medical Center, Nashville, TN, USA

M. C. Shinall Jr (✉)
Department of Surgery, Vanderbilt University Medical Center, Nashville, TN, USA
e-mail: ricky.shinall@vumc.org

© Springer Nature Switzerland AG 2022
D. A. Edwards et al. (eds.), *Hospitalized Chronic Pain Patient*,
https://doi.org/10.1007/978-3-031-08376-1_26

Management of the pain itself requires administering analgesic agents based on the patient's history of analgesic use and the nature and intensity of the patient's current pain. The patient's life-limiting disease will often limit the available options or routes of administration, as in this case of malignant bowel obstruction that required parenteral opioids until the nausea was adequately managed and the patient could resume oral intake.

Although the patient's disease can tie the pain specialist's hands in a number of ways, the patient's short life-expectancy frees the physician to treat pain without worries about long-term sequelae of treatment. Specifically, opioids can be aggressively up-titrated to control pain without concern for long-term dependence. Some have expressed concern that aggressive escalation of opioids for treatment of terminally ill patients may shorten patients' lives. However, the evidence shows that aggressive titration of opioids for symptoms does not hasten death [1].

Just as they do to treat any other type of pain, physicians treating a patient with short life expectancy should try to identify a treatable cause of pain. The patient's limited prognosis might make certain treatments inadvisable, but other less invasive procedures might remain possibilities. In this case, although definitive surgical treatment of the bowel obstruction was not possible, the surgeon was still able to alleviate symptoms with a less invasive procedure via a gastrostomy [2]. Whenever a pathologic process is identified causing the pain, a specialist in treating that process should be consulted to determine whether any intervention is possible. Such specialists include radiation oncologists, endoscopists, interventional pain specialists, and surgeons.

If available, a multidisciplinary palliative care team can help the patient navigate the issues at the end of life [3]. A short life expectancy can cause distress in several ways. Patients may worry that pain or other symptoms will increase as death approaches. Some patients may have profound spiritual crises as they face their own mortality. Other patients may have concerns about how their families will manage without them. The distress of families about the impending loss of their loved one can also cause the patient distress. Multidisciplinary palliative care teams combine multiple professionals who can help patients at the end of life. If a dedicated palliative care team is not available, the treating physician may need to discern what about the patient's impending death is causing the most distress to determine what other professionals may help the patient. Psychologists can help if the patient has poor coping strategies. Chaplains are most helpful dealing with spiritual distress. Social workers can help the patient navigate the interpersonal relationships and social issues that cause them distress. Unless these forms of distress are alleviated, the treating physician will find it extremely difficult to manage the patient's pain. We have seen frequent examples in our experience of pain medication dosing and frequency requirements decrease after these "total pain" issues are addressed and mitigated.

Patients with limited life expectancy will often be eligible for hospice benefits, which provide excellent resources for managing pain. Hospice is an insurance benefit under Medicare and most other forms of insurance that provides visits by nurses, nurses' aides, social workers, chaplains, and volunteers to patients with limited life expectancy. Hospice also provides bereavement support to family members after the patient's death. To be eligible for hospice, a patient must have a life expectancy of 6 months or less in the opinion of two physicians, but the benefits can be continued indefinitely as long as the patient is expected to die within a 6-month period. Patients must also be willing to forego disease-modifying therapy to enroll in hospice. Hospice benefits can be delivered to patients in their homes or in facilities, and inpatient hospice care is available for patients whose symptom burden requires skilled nursing to manage [4].

Because enrolling in hospice means foregoing further life-prolonging care for their condition, many patients are resistant to the idea and many physicians are reluctant to discuss it. Nevertheless, the interdisciplinary hospice team can be a powerful resource to help manage the patient's total pain, and it should be offered to patients who would qualify for it. Many hospice agencies will provide informational visits to help patients and their families decide if hospice is right for them.

The pain specialist treating a patient who is likely to enroll in hospice should keep this fact in mind in developing a treatment plan for pain. Hospice agencies receive a capitated per diem payment to provide all medical care for enrolled patients, and so most hospices are not financially capable of providing very expensive therapies. Cost should therefore be a consideration in developing a treatment plan for a patient who is likely to be enrolled in hospice.

References

1. Portenoym RK, et al. Opioid use and survival at the end of life: a survey of a hospice population. J Pain Symptom Manag. 2006;32(6):532–40.
2. Thomay AA, Jaques DP, Miner TJ. Surgical palliative care: getting back to our roots. Surg Clin N Am. 2009;81(1):27–41.
3. Saunders C. The evolution of palliative care. Patient Educ Couns. 2000;41(3):7–13.
4. Gazelle G. Understanding hospice—an underutilized option for life's final chapter. N Engl J Med. 2007;357(4):321–4.

Case 17: Management of a Pain/Dyspnea in an Actively Dying Patient

27

Bethany-Rose Daubman

Key Points

- For patients who have previously been on opioids, they should be continued in the last hours/days of life, even if no observable pain is present [1].
- Many patients are unable to take PO at the end of life and have fluctuating symptom management issues which may be best addressed with IV or subcutaneous opioids. It is often recommended to convert PO medications to IV (bolus +/− infusion) in these cases [2].
- However, actively dying patients should only be on a continuous infusion of opioids if they have symptoms that are best treated by opioids (pain or dyspnea) and have had frequent PRN opioid requirements.
- Opioid continuous infusions should not be increased more than every 8 h (the time required to reach steady state). The hourly continuous infusion rate can be increased based on the total amount of boluses required in the previous 8 h, divided by 8 to determine the additional hourly rate required.
- Always treat acute pain or dyspnea with boluses, not through increasing the basal rate of a continuous infusion, as this will take time to reach steady state and will not immediately address the distress.
- There is no evidence that opioids hasten death when administered properly at the end of life [3].
- Treatment and care plan is outlined below in Fig. 27.1.

B.-R. Daubman (✉)
Division of Palliative Care and Geriatrics, Department of Medicine, Massachusetts General Hospital, Harvard University, Boston, MA, USA
e-mail: bdaubman@partners.org

© Springer Nature Switzerland AG 2022
D. A. Edwards et al. (eds.), *Hospitalized Chronic Pain Patient*,
https://doi.org/10.1007/978-3-031-08376-1_27

Assess symptoms and select appropriate medications and routes	• Mrs. Valdez is likely experiencing pain secondary to her hip fracture. She is also likely experiencing dyspnea secondary to her pneumonia. • You decide that both her pain and dyspnea can be best treated with an opioid, and you decide on morphine, which has worked well for her in the past.
Convert oral opioids into IV or subcutaneous route if needed	• Mrs. Valdez is no longer able to take PO, so you decide to convert her morphine from PO to IV (basal and bolus dosing). • She was using a total of 115mg PO morphine per day (40mg in long acting, and 75mg in short acting morphine), which is equivalent to ~38mg IV morphine (3:1 conversion ratio). • Start a morphine continuous infusion at 1.5mg/hr (38mg/24hr= ~1.5mg/hr).
Select appropriate bolus dosing and intervals	• Bolus dosing should be ~50-150% of the continuous rate, and can be titrated up as the continuous rate is increased. • For Mrs. Valdez, as you are worried about her currently untreated pain and dyspnea, you start with a bolus of 2mg IV morphine q 30 minutes prn pain or dyspnea.
Adjust continuous infusion based on PRN requirements	• Over the next 8 hours, Mrs. Valdez requires 10mg IV morphine in prn dosing, and appears less dyspneic and uncomfortable after receiving the boluses. • You divide 10mg/8 hours to increase the continuous rate by 1mg/hr. • Her new continuous infusion rate is now 2.5mg/hr, and you increase her morphine bolus dosing to 2-4mg q 30 minutes PRN.
Counsel family on symptom management at end of life	• Mrs. Valdez's son is glad she appears more comfortable now, but expresses concern. "I don't want to see her suffer, but I don't want the pain medication to end her life." • You reassure him that you will only use medications to treat her symptoms, not to shorten her life. He is comforted to hear research has shown that when given this way, morphine does not hasten death.

Fig. 27.1 Treatment and care plan

Outcome

Mrs. Valdez's pain and tachypnea improved with up-titration of her morphine continuous infusion to 2.5 mg/h. She became less responsive, but occasionally would open her eyes when family squeezed her hands. She still occasionally moaned and became tachypneic with any repositioning, so you continued to up-titrate her basal rate of morphine based on her bolus requirements. Her family feels comfortable with the plan of care, saying, "We're glad she's not moaning anymore, and we know you're doing everything you can to make sure she's comfortable as she's dying." The next day, Mrs. Valdez dies peacefully surrounded by her family.

References

1. Mori M, Elsayem A, Reddy SK, Bruera E, Fadul NA. Unrelieved pain and suffering in patients with advanced cancer. Am J Hosp Palliat Care. 2012;29(3):236–40.
2. Ryan H, Schofield P, Bowman D, et al. How to recognize and manage psychological distress in cancer patients. Eur J Cancer Care. 2005;14(1):7–15.
3. Ellershaw J, Ward C. Care of the dying patient: the last hours or days of life. BMJ. 2003;326(7379):30–4.

Part IV

Medication Treatments

Opioids

28

Daltry Dott and Christopher M. Sobey

Common Opioids

Pain is the most common symptom for which patients present to a physician. Patients with chronic pain may present to the hospital with increased, breakthrough, or new acute on chronic pain complaints that need to be managed during admission to the hospital. Multiple opioids are available for pain treatment and have differing routes of administration, dosages, half-lives and special considerations (Table 28.1).

Patients who lack enteral access may require IV or transdermal opioids until enteral access is available. After enteral access is available, 24-h IV and/or transdermal opioid requirements should be calculated, and the patient should be transitioned to PO opioids (see "Opioid Conversion" below).

Opioid Cross-Tolerance

Cross-tolerance occurs when tolerance to the effects of one drug produces tolerance to another drug. This can allow a patient to have tolerance to a drug that he or she has never used before. Incomplete cross-tolerance can cause a greater than anticipated potency in a new opioid. When converting from one opioid to another, the opioid dose should be reduced by 25–50% to accommodate for unknown cross-tolerance. There is a wide variation among individuals that is multifactorial and poorly understood.

D. Dott
Department of Anesthesiology, University of Texas Southwestern, Dallas, TX, USA

C. M. Sobey (✉)
Department of Anesthesiology, Vanderbilt University Medical Center, Nashville, TN, USA
e-mail: christopher.m.sobey@vumc.org

© Springer Nature Switzerland AG 2022
D. A. Edwards et al. (eds.), *Hospitalized Chronic Pain Patient*,
https://doi.org/10.1007/978-3-031-08376-1_28

Table 28.1 Common opioids [1]

Opioid	Route of administration	Common doses	Half-life (DOA)	Special considerations
Morphine (natural)	IV[a]	4–15 mg q3–4 h	2.5–3 h (3–7 h)	– Caution in renal failure
	IM	2.5–20 mg q3–4 h		– Active metabolite morphine-6-glucuronide can lead to increased sedation
	SQ	2.5–20 mg q3–4 h		– Causes histamine release
	PO			
	– ER	15–200 mg q8–12 h		
	– IR	5–30 mg q3–4 h		
	SL	5–30 mg q3–4 h		
	Buccal	5–30 mg q3–4 h		
	IT[a]	0.2–1 mg one time dose		
	Epidural[a]	2–10 mg one time dose		
	PR	10–30 mg q4 h		
Codeine (natural)	IV	30–60 mg q4–6 h	2.5–3 h (4–6 h)	– Codeine must be metabolized by hepatic CYP2D6 to morphine for analgesic effect. Pain relief may be inadequate in individuals who are poor metabolizers. Ultra-rapid metabolizers may experience symptoms of overdose (sleepiness, confusion, altered breathing)
	IM	30–60 mg q4–6 h		
	SQ	30–60 mg q4–6 h		
	PO			
Oxycodone (semisynthetic)	PO		(3–6 h)	
	– ER	5–15 mg q4–6 h	4.5 h	
	– IR	10–640 mg q12 h	2–3 h	

Table 28.1   (continued)

Opioid	Route of administration	Common doses	Half-life (DOA)	Special considerations
Oxymorphone (semisynthetic)	IV	0.5 mg q4–6 h	7–9 h	
	PO			
	– ER	5–40 mg q12 h	(12 h)	
	– IR	5–40 mg q4–6 h	(4–6 h)	
	IM	5–10 mg q12 h		
	SQ	1–1.5 mg q4–6 h		
	PR	1–1.5 mg q4–6 h		
	IN			
Hydromorphone (semisynthetic)	IV	0.2–1 mg q4 h	2–3 h	
	IM	1–2 mg q2–3 h	(4–6 h)	
	PO			
	– ER	8–32 mg daily		
	– IR	2–4 mg q4–6 h		
	PR	3 mg q6–8 h		
Hydrocodone (semisynthetic)	PO		3–4 h	
	– ER	10–100 mg q12 h	(4–8 h)	
	– IR	5–10 mg q4–6 h		
Buprenorphine (semisynthetic)	IV	0.3 mg q6 h	24–37 h	– Very high affinity for mu-receptor. Patients may need very high doses of other, stronger opioids to displace buprenorphine from the mu-receptors and provide adequate pain relief
	IM	0.3 mg q6 h	(6 h)	
	SL	4–24 mg q24 h		
	TD			
	SD	4 implants with 74.2 mg in each		

(continued)

Table 28.1 (continued)

Opioid	Route of administration	Common doses	Half-life (DOA)	Special considerations
Nalbuphine (semisynthetic)	IV	10–20 mg q3–6 h	3–6 h	
	IM	10–20 mg q3–6 h	(3–6 h)	
	SQ	10–20 mg q3–6 h		
Methadone (synthetic)	IV	2.5–10 mg q8–12 h	7–65 h (single dose: 4–8 h; prolonged use: 1–2 days)	– Long and variable half-life when administered PO
	PO	2.5–20 mg q8–24 h		– Also an NMDA receptor antagonist
Fentanyl (synthetic)	IV[a]	25–100 mg	10–20 m	– Highly lipophilic, very long context sensitive half life
	IN	1.5 µg/kg	6.5 m	
	SL	100–800 µg q2 h	5–6 h	
	Buccal	100–800 µg q2 h	5–6 h	
	Lollipop	200 µg q4 h	5–6 h	
	TD	25–100 µg/h q72 h	20–27 h (30–60 m)	
Sufentanil (synthetic)	IV[a]	1–2 µg/kg	160 m (30–60 m)	
Remifentanil (synthetic)	IV[a]	0.5–1 µg/kg	1–20 m (5–10 m)	– Rapidly metabolized by nonspecific esterases
Tramadol (synthetic)	PO		5–7 h	
	– ER	100–300 mg daily		– Weak mu-receptor agonist
	– IR	25–100 mg q4–6 h		– NE and 5HT reuptake inhibitor
Meperidine (synthetic)	IV[a]	25–100 mg q4 h	2.5–4 h	– Potentially fatal interaction with MAOIs
	IM	25–100 mg q4 h		– Metabolite normeperidine can accumulate in renal failure and cause neuroexcitation (seizures)
	PO	50–100 mg q4 h		– Can be used to treat postoperative shivering

Table 28.1 (continued)

Opioid	Route of administration	Common doses	Half-life (DOA)	Special considerations
Tapentadol (synthetic)	PO		4 h	– Decreases the seizure threshold
	– ER	50–250 mg q12 h		
	– IR	50–100 mg q4–6 h		

IV intravenous, *IM* intramuscular, *SQ* subcutaneous, *PO* oral, *ER* extended release, *IR* immediate relief, *SL* sublingual, *IT* intrathecal, *PR* rectal, *IN* intranasal, *TD* transdermal, *SD* subdermal implant, *DOA* duration of action, *h* hours, *m* minutes, *mg* milligram, *q* every, *d* day
[a]Can also be given as a continuous infusion or used as patient controlled anesthesia (PCA)

Table 28.2 Opioid conversion [2]

Drug	Conversion factor to morphine	Conversion factor from morphine	Equianalgesic dose IM/IV (mg)	PO (mg)
Morphine	1	1	10	30
Hydromorphone	×5	1/5	1.5	7.5
Oxycodone	×1.5	1/1.5	–	20
Hydrocodone	×1	×1	–	30
Fentanyl	×100	1/100	–	0.1
Codeine	/10	×10	130	200
Nalbuphine	×1	×1		
Oxymorphone	×3	1/3	1	10
Tapentadol	×1	×1		
Tramadol	/10	×10	100	120
Buprenorphine	×10	1/10	0.3	0.4 (SL)
Meperidine	/10	×10	100	300
Methadone	–[a]	–[a]	1	2

[a]See conversion for methadone in Table 28.3

Opioid Conversion

When a patient is being treated with chronic opioids and they present to the hospital with acute pain, determining their new daily opioid requirement may be difficult. Starting patient-controlled analgesia (PCA) with an opioid, such as hydromorphone or morphine, can help determine a patient's 24-h opioid needs, which can then be converted to oral equivalents (Tables 28.2, 28.3 and 28.4).

How to convert PCA (IV) dosing to PO

1. Convert the total 24-h IV opioid needs to morphine equivalents.

   (a) 24-h IV opioid use multiplied or divided by the conversion factor to morphine in Table 28.2.

Table 28.3 Methadone conversion [3]

24 h Oral morphine usage (mg)	Oral morphine:methadone ratio
<30	2:1
31–99	4:1
100–299	8:1
300–499	12:1
500–999	15:1
1000–1200	20:1
>1200	Consider consult

Table 28.4 Opioid patch to oral morphine conversion [4]

Drug	Patch strength (µg/h)	PO morphine dose
Buprenorphine	5	15 mg/24 h
Fentanyl	12	30–45 mg/24 h

2. Choose an oral agent to be used and convert the morphine equivalents to the chosen agent.

   (a) 24-h morphine equivalent usage multiplied or divided by the conversion factor from morphine in Table 28.2.
3. Decrease the new dose by at least 25–30% (up to 50%) to allow for incomplete cross-tolerance.
4. Divide total daily dose by the number of times to be given per day, commonly q4–6 h.

   (a) If starting a patient on a long-acting agent, it is recommended to divide the total daily opioid needs in half and give one half as long-acting split into two doses per day (q12 h) and the other half split throughout the day (q4–6 h) for breakthrough pain.

Opioid Metabolites

Different opioids have different metabolites. Urine drug screens can be used to determine compliance, misuse, diversion, or recreational use (Fig. 28.1).

Opioid Rotation

After initiation and titration of opioids, the initial clinical efficacy may gradually decline, or increased doses may produce undesirable side effects. It is unclear why opioid rotation improves the analgesic effect, although cross-tolerance seems to play a role. It is believed that alterations in the binding to µ-opioid receptors affects patients differently, and the effect of opioid rotation is related to the incomplete cross-tolerance of opioids [6]. Switching opioids has been shown to result in improvement in >50% of patients with chronic pain who do not initially respond to one opioid or have

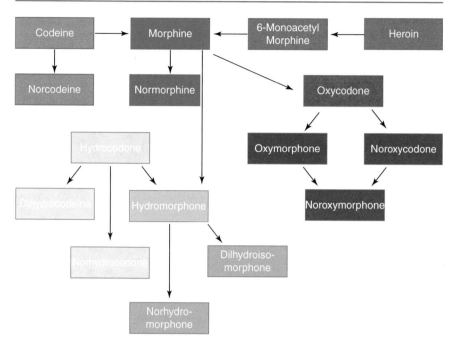

Fig. 28.1 Opioid metabolites [5]

intolerable side effects [7]. Opioid rotation may allow for improved pain control, lower doses of medication, increased efficacy, and decreased side-effects.

Opioid rotation conversion
1. Calculate 24-h dose in morphine equivalents
2. Convert to second opioid
3. Reduce dose by at least 25–30% to account for incomplete cross-tolerance
4. Divide into an appropriate dosing schedule

Opioid Addiction

Patients who present with opioid abuse/addiction should be referred to addiction psychiatry for rehabilitation and detoxification.

References

1. Cherny NI. The pharmacologic management of cancer pain. Oncology. 2004;18(12):1499–515.
2. McPherson ML. Demystifying opioid conversion calculations: a guide for effective dosing. Bethesda: ASHP; 2010.
3. Wong E, Walker K. A review of common methods to convert morphine to methadone. J Community Hosp Intern Med Perspect. 2012;2(4):19541.

4. Vartan CM. Buprenorphine transdermal patch: an overview for use in chronic pain. US Pharm. 2014;39(10):HS16–20.
5. Gourlay D, Heit H, Caplan Y. Urine drug testing in primary care: dispelling the myths and designing strategies. Monogr Calif Acad Fam Physicians. 2002;27(3):260–7.
6. Pasternak GW. Incomplete cross tolerance and multiple mu opioid peptide receptors. Trends Pharmacol Sci. 2001;22:67–70.
7. Mercadante S, Bruera E. Opioid switching: a systematic and critical review. Cancer Treat Rev. 2006;32(4):304–15.

Nonsteroidal Anti-Inflammatory Drugs (NSAIDs)

29

Christopher M. Sobey

Background

NSAIDs function through the inhibition of the cyclooxygenase (COX) enzymes, which are responsible for catalyzing the formation of prostaglandin precursors (prostanoids). Prostaglandin formation of PGD_2, PGE_2, PGF_2, PGI_2 (prostacyclin), and thromboxane A2 (TXA_2) is thereby inhibited, which has an array of downstream effects. Prostanoids have both central and peripheral mechanisms that can increase neural excitability, reduce pain thresholds and potentiate pain pathways, thus inhibiting production of these mediators is the primary analgesic mechanism of NSAIDs [1]. In the peripheral nervous system, prostaglandins regulate sensitivity of nociceptors (A-delta and C-fibers) resulting in a cascade of events that hypopolarize the neurons, increasing stimulation and transmission. In the central nervous system, prostaglandins increase concentration of pro-nociceptive neurotransmitters such as Substance P and glutamate, increase the sensitivity of second order neurons, and decrease the release of inhibitory neurotransmitters such as glycine.

There are two major cyclooxygenase enzymes (COX-1 and 2) that are responsible for the variable effects of prostanoids/prostaglandins. COX-1 is constitutively (continually) expressed, where as COX-2 is induced by presence of inflammatory mediators. COX-1 expression has downstream effects on gastrointestinal protection, platelet activity, renal function, and tissue inflammation, whereas COX-2 effects are more selective for just tissue inflammation and renal function. The beneficial and detrimental results of various COX inhibitors frequently will depend on the ratio of selectivity of COX-1 and 2 inhibition.

C. M. Sobey (✉)
Department of Anesthesiology, Vanderbilt University Medical Center, Nashville, TN, USA
e-mail: christopher.m.sobey@vumc.org

© Springer Nature Switzerland AG 2022
D. A. Edwards et al. (eds.), *Hospitalized Chronic Pain Patient*,
https://doi.org/10.1007/978-3-031-08376-1_29

Types of NSAIDs

Traditional NSAIDs inhibit both COX-1 and 2 enzymes, with varying degrees of selectivity. COX-2 selective inhibitors have very little effect on inhibition of COX-1. Generally, the efficacy of analgesia comparing traditional to COX-2 selective inhibitors is fairly equivalent overall. Primary benefit of selective COX-2 inhibitors is to minimize GI side effects associated with use. The COX-2 inhibitors rofecoxib (Vioxx) and valdecoxib (Bextra) were both withdrawn from US market due to "potential increased risk for serious cardiovascular adverse events." Please see Table 29.1 for details on types and dosing.

Benefits

- Nonsteroidal anti-inflammatory drugs can be effectively used as a primary analgesic as well as to supplement the use of other analgesics, such as opioids, to provide a heightened degree of pain relief. Opioid dose reduction has been demonstrated when NSAIDs are used in combination, with trials producing between 30–50% sparing effect on morphine consumption. This sparing effect also results in reduction of opioid-based side effects such as postoperative nausea and vomiting

Table 29.1 NSAIDs

Name	Type	Dose	Max	Notes
Ibuprofen (Advil, Motrin)	Traditional	400–800 mg q6-8h	3200 mg/day	*Racemic mixture, only (+)S isomer is active, (−R) isomer is inactive but can be converted to (−)S isomer.*
Naproxen (Aleve)	Traditional	250–500 mg PO q12h	1500 mg/day	*May have the least cardiovascular risk of all NSAIDs*
Meloxicam (Mobic)	Traditional	7.5–15 mg daily	15 mg/day	*No need for dose adjustments in patients with mild to moderate renal impairment*
Diclofenac (Voltaren, Solaraze)	Traditional	50 mg PO q8-12h or 75 mg q12h. XR form available at 100 mg daily, IV: 37.5 mg q6h Topical (1% and 3% formulations)	150 mg/day	*Multiple routes of administration (PO, IV, topical, transdermal patch) Can be combined with misoprostol (Arthrotec) to reduce GI side effects*
Ketorolac (Toradol)	Traditional	15–30 mg IM/IV q6h 10 mg q4-6h	120 mg/day IV 40 mg/day PO	*BBW – short term (up to 5d); Increased serious GI adverse event risk; contraindicated in patients with adv. Renal disease or increased bleeding risk*
Celecoxib (Celebrex)	COX-2 Selective	50–200 mg po daily or BID	400 mg/day	*Only COX-2 selective inhibitor available on market in US*

(PONV) and sedation by 30% and 29% respectively. Due to this opioid-sparing effect there is a theoretical reduction in urinary retention, pruritus, and respiratory depression with concomitant NSAID use, however studies have not demonstrated a significant effect on these outcomes. Multiple studies have demonstrated benefits with the addition of perioperative NSAIDs as part of a balance analgesic treatment plan in an array of surgical procedures. This resulted in improved pain scores, decreased opioid requirement, greater hemodynamic stability, ability to participate in recovery protocols, and higher Global Evaluation ratings.

Adverse Effects

There are limitations on the utility of NSAIDs for certain patients. Specific adverse effects related to these drugs need to be appreciated and monitored for, with individual patient factors often precluding the appropriateness of use due to safety concerns.

- Gastropathy

  - Gastric protection is mediated by PGI2 and PGE2, which produce an increase in bicarbonate and mucous production, increase in blood flow, and decrease H+ secretion. NSAIDs suppress release of prostaglandins, thus inhibiting these mechanisms and increasing the risk of ulceration [2].
  - This is not uncommon, with between 15–30% of chronic users having an effect on gastric mucosa on EGD. Patients with ulcerations often will be without symptoms, with "silent" ulceration in as many as 70% of users.
  - As many as 25% of chronic NSAID users develop ulcer disease and 2–4% will bleed or perforate
  - Studies comparing non-selective and selective NSAIDs demonstrate that COX-2 selective medications have been shown to be less irritating to GI mucosa, producing fewer incidents of abdominal discomfort, gastritis, ulcerations. Schnitzer, et al. in the TARGET study concluded that use of lumiracoxib was associated with a threefold to fourfold reduction in serious GI complications compared to traditional NSAIDs, and Bombardier, et al. in the VIGOR study showed a 50% relative risk reduction for GI complications when using rofecoxib compared to naproxen.

- Nephrotoxicity

  - Multiple studies have illuminated the potential consequence of acute kidney injury with use of NSAIDs [3]. If has been postulated that this injury occurs from both hemodynamic alterations as well as acute interstitial nephritis. In most healthy individuals, prostaglandins do not play a major role in renal blood flow, however in patients with either pre-existing conditions or acute stresses that result in prolonged renal vasoconstriction, prostaglandin-mediated afferent arteriole vasodilation helps compensate in these low flow

states and increases renal perfusion. When PG synthesis is compromised with use of NSAID, this compensatory mechanism is impaired, thus resulting in reduced renal blood flow and glomerular filtration rate due to increased preglomerular resistance.
- The theoretical adverse effects on renal dysfunction appear to be primarily associated with COX-1 inhibition. Multiple meta-analyses performed comparing COX-1 and 2 have demonstrated that the pooled risk ratios of COX-2 selective NSAIDs were less than that of traditional NSAIDs, however did not reach statistical significance.

- Platelet dysfunction

  - Inhibition of cyclooxygenase enzymes present in platelets results in blocking formation of thromboxane A2, which acts as both a vasoconstrictor and platelet aggregator. Inhibition of this process by NSAIDs can increase bleeding propensity and bleeding time. Use of aspirin has demonstrated increased risk of spontaneous hematomas and post-surgical bleeding that can lead to complications [4]. Studies have demonstrated this risk of intra-operative and post-operative bleeding has not been significantly increased with COX-2 selective inhibitors, as they do not exert significant effect on platelet function. Nonselective NSAIDs, most notably ketorolac, has demonstrated a greater effect on platelet aggregation inhibition and use should be risk-stratified.

- Osteogenesis

  - Prolonged administration of nonsteroidal anti-inflammatory medications has been demonstrated to interfere with osteogenesis, as cytokine inhibition can impair chemotaxis of inflammatory cells and the downstream cascade of bone matrix synthesis [5]. However, short-term use of both traditional NSAIDs and COX-2 selective inhibitors has been determined to be safe in the setting of primary bone healing and callous formation. A retrospective review performed by Blomquist, et al., confirmed that short-term postoperative treatment with NSAIDs did not have a negative influence on functional outcome measures after arthroscopic Bankart procedures. Use of NSAIDs should be reconsidered in patients who demonstrate other risk factors of delayed fracture healing, or if a fracture demonstrates evidence of delayed union.

- Cardiovascular Risks

  - Studies have demonstrated increased risk of cardiovascular events with use of both traditional and selective COX-2 inhibitors, with increased risk of thrombotic events, atrial tachyarrhythmias, and ventricular tachyarrhythmias. The most commonly accepted mechanism relating to an imbalance in vasoconstrictive and pro-aggregatory effects of thromboxane (TXA2) and the vasodilating and anti-aggregatory effects of PGI_2 [6]. Selective COX-2 inhibitors have a greater effect on this imbalance, leaving the COX-1 derived thromboxane effect intact, thus increasing risk of vaso-occlusive events [7]. There is evidence that sparing inhibition of PGI_2 will in fact reduce the risk of CV adverse events. An alternative proposed mechanism accounting for the increasing cardiovascular risk with nonsteroidal agents related to the reduced oxygen free radical antioxidant capacity that can result in accumulation of oxidized LDL.

- Non-selective NSAIDs have been determined to be safer in regards to cardiovascular events due to the aforementioned mechanism, an example of which being rofecoxib (Vioxx) which was withdrawn from the market in 2004 due to higher risk of event occurance.
- All nonsteroidal anti-inflammatory drugs have been determined to have some increase in cardiovascular events; however traditional nonselective COX inhibitors demonstrate less risk than selective COX-2 [8]. The degree of risk with traditional NSAIDs appears to be related to the ratio of COX-2 inhibition relative to COX-1. Traditional NSAIDs ibuprofen and naproxen were noted to be the least likely to increase risk of cardiovascular events, with relative risk values close to 1 in multiple studies. In calculating relative risk reduction across multiple reviews, naproxen had a significantly lower risk than ibuprofen. The greatest risk of CV events was with rofecoxib (discontinued), celecoxib, and diclofenac.

References

1. Bingham S, Beswick PJ, Blum DE, Gray NM, Chessell IP. The role of cyclooxygenase pathway in nociception and pain. Semin Cell Dev Biol. 2006;17(5):544–54.
2. Bombardier C, Laine L, Reicin A, Shapiro D, Burgos-Vargas R, Davis B, et al. Comparison of upper gastrointestinal toxicity of rofecoxib and naproxen in patients with rheumatoid arthritis. VIGOR study group. N Engl J Med. 2000;343:1520–8.
3. Ungprasert P, Cheungpasitporn W, Crowson CS, Matteson EL. Individual non-steroidal anti-inflammatory drugs and risk of acute kidney injury: a systematic review and meta-analysis of observational studies. Eur J Intern Med. 2015;26(4):285–91.
4. Schafer AI. Effects of nonsteroidal anti-inflammatory drugs on platelet function and systemic hemostasis. J Clin Pharmacol. 1995;35:209–19.
5. Giannoudis PV, Hak D, Sanders D, Donohoe E, Tosounidis T, Bahney C. Inflammation, bone healing, and anti-inflammatory drugs: an update. J Orthop Trauma. 2015;29(Suppl 12):S6–9.
6. Trelle S, Reichenbach S, Wandel S, et al. Cardiovascular safety of non-steroidal anti-inflammatory drugs: network meta-analysis. BMJ. 2011;342:c7086.
7. Gerstein NS, Gerstein WH, Carey MC, et al. The thrombotic and arrhythmogenic risks of perioperative NSAIDs. J Cardiothorac Vasc Anesth. 2014;28(2):369–78.
8. Solomon SD, McMurray JJV, Pfeffer MA, Wittes J, Fowler R, Finn P, et al. Cardiovascular risk associated with celecoxib in a clinical trial for colorectal adenoma prevention. N Engl J Med. 2005;352:1071–80.

Acetaminophen

30

David A. Edwards and Obi Okwuchukwu

Mechanism of Action

The MOA of acetaminophen is not fully understood. It is believed to act centrally, inhibiting the synthesis of prostaglandins by blocking the activity of cyclooxygenase-1 and cyclooxygenase-2 [1]. This mechanism appears primarily central in nature, with weak anti-inflammatory actions in the periphery. For this reason, many of the adverse effects of typical NSAIDs such as GI intolerance and platelet function are fairly limited with acetaminophen.

Administration

Acetaminophen can be administered orally, rectally and intravenously.

Dosage

The maximum daily dose for acetaminophen is 4 g for an adult as recommended by the FDA. A decreased dose (2–3 g daily) is recommended for patients with chronic liver disease [2].

Acetaminophen is commonly combined with opioids and other over-the-counter medications, and care must be taken during medication reconciliation to account for all sources of acetaminophen.

D. A. Edwards
Departments of Anesthesiology and Neurological Surgery, Vanderbilt University Medical Center, Nashville, TN, USA
e-mail: david.a.edwards@vumc.org

O. Okwuchukwu (✉)
Las Vegas Pain Institute, Las Vegas, NV, USA
e-mail: oobi@lvpimedical.com

© Springer Nature Switzerland AG 2022
D. A. Edwards et al. (eds.), *Hospitalized Chronic Pain Patient*,
https://doi.org/10.1007/978-3-031-08376-1_30

Acetaminophen is a helpful adjunct to reduce the required doses of other agents, such as opioids, and avoidance of opioid-related adverse events. Both PO and IV formulations have demonstrated improvement in post-operative analgesia, with intravenous administration demonstrating superior rapid-onset relief compared to by mouth administration [3, 4]. Dosed at 1 g q6 hours, IV acetaminophen usage resulted in 33% reduction in morphine consumption over 24 h in orthopedic surgeries, as well as reduced need for rescue medication.

Acetaminophen is currently the leading cause of acute liver failure in the United States. Hepatotoxicity usually results from excessive intake of acetaminophen [5]. There is increased risk for patients with history of alcoholism or chronic hepatitis.

For hospitalized patients who will require opioids and acetaminophen for pain management, it is recommended that both drugs be separated and adjusted independently to ensure that total daily dose from all sources be accounted for. It is also prudent to ensure that medication administration is properly documented to avoid double dosing or early dosing when acetaminophen is ordered on a PRN basis.

Contraindications

There are relatively few contraindications to acetaminophen and include allergy to acetaminophen. Patients with chronic liver disease should be treated with a decreased dose as mentioned above [6].

References

1. Botting RM. Mechanism of action of acetaminophen: is there a cyclooxygenase 3? Clin Infect Dis. 2000;31(Suppl 5):S202–10.
2. Chandok N, Watt KD. Pain management in the cirrhotic patient: the clinical challenge. Mayo Clin Proc. 2010;85(5):451–8.
3. Ennis ZN, et al. Acetaminophen for chronic pain: a systematic review on efficacy. Basic Clin Pharmacol Toxicol. 2016;118(3):184–9.
4. Wick EC, Grant MC, Wu CL. Postoperative multimodal analgesia pain management with non-opioid analgesics and techniques: a review. JAMA Surg. 2017;52(7):691–7.
5. Lewis JH, Stine JG. Review article: prescribing medications in patients with cirrhosis - a practical guide. Aliment Pharmacol Ther. 2013;37(12):1132–56.
6. Moore RA, et al. Overview review: comparative efficacy of oral ibuprofen and paracetamol (acetaminophen) across acute and chronic pain conditions. Eur J Pain. 2015;19(9):1213–23.

Local Anesthetics

31

Jeff A. Gartner and Brian F. S. Allen

What Are Local Anesthetics?

Local anesthetic (LA) molecules are composed of an aromatic ring linked to a tertiary amine via either an ester or amide linkage. This linkage is used to categorize LAs as either aminoesters or aminoamides (hereafter called esters and amides). By convention, the names of amide LAs have 2 "i's" (lidocaine, ropivacaine) while ester LAs have one "i" (procaine, tetracaine). Variations in the aromatic or tertiary amine structures between LAs result in differences in physiochemical properties such as pKa, hydrophobicity, and protein binding that alter onset, duration, and clearance among local anesthetics (Table 31.1).

Mechanism of Action

Local anesthetics prevent axonal signal transduction by voltage-gated sodium channels (VGSC) blockade, interfering with sodium influx and preventing depolarization. VGSCs exist in 3 functional states (resting, activated, and inactivated). LAs bind the intracellular aspect of the VGSC with greater affinity for the activated and inactivated states (compared to resting state). This means LA onset is most rapid and profound on neurons that are firing [1]. Neuron size (diameter) and myelination also affect susceptibility to conduction blockade. Small, myelinated fibers are most susceptible, followed by large myelinated fibers. Unmyelinated, small C fibers are the most resistant to conduction blockade. Some local anesthetics, notably

J. A. Gartner
Department of Anesthesiology, Ascension Medical Group, Nashville, TN, USA

B. F. S. Allen (✉)
Department of Anesthesiology, Vanderbilt University Medical Center, Nashville, TN, USA
e-mail: brian.allen@vumc.org

© Springer Nature Switzerland AG 2022
D. A. Edwards et al. (eds.), *Hospitalized Chronic Pain Patient*,
https://doi.org/10.1007/978-3-031-08376-1_31

Table 31.1 Local Anesthetic Properties [1–3]

Amide LAs	pKa	Lipophilicity (partition coefficient)	Protein binding	Potency	Maximum recommended LA dose	Maximum LA dose with epinephrine	Elimination half life (hours)
Mepivacaine	7.72	130	Moderate	Low	5 mg/kg (400 mg max)	7 mg/kg (500 mg max)	1.9
Lidocaine	7.76	366	Moderate	Low	5 mg/kg (300 mg max)	7 mg/kg (500 mg max)	1.6
Ropivacaine	8.16	775	High	High	2.5 mg/kg (225 mg max)	2.5 mg/kg (225 mg max)	1.9
Bupivacaine	8.10	3420	High	High	2.5 mg/kg (200 mg max)	2.5 mg/kg (200 mg max)	3.5
Ester Las							
2-Chlorprocaine	9.06	810	N/A	Low	10 mg/kg (800 mg max)	14 mg/kg (1000 mg max)	0.11
Procaine	8.89	100	Low	Low	7 mg/kg	10 mg/kg	0.14
Tetracaine	8.38	5822	High	High	1 mg/kg	1.5 mg/kg	1.25

ropivacaine, demonstrate selectivity for sensory (over motor) nerves, though at high concentrations they result in motor blockade.

Local anesthetics can be administered via a number of routes, including perineural, neuraxial, transdermal, oral, intravenous, and subcutaneous (as wound infiltration or surgical tumescence).

Pharmacokinetics

Metabolism

Ester and amide LAs are cleared from the body in different ways: esters via ester hydrolysis by plasma cholinesterases, amides via liver P-450 enzymes. True allergic reactions are rare, but more likely with ester LAs than amides. A reported allergy should be investigated since it may represent allergy to a preservative, a non-allergic symptom (e.g., tachycardia from epinephrine administered with LA for dental work), or a manifestation of local anesthetic systemic toxicity (LAST). When allergy to an ester LA does occur, it safe to give amide LAs.

Local anesthetic potency is affected by lipid solubility. Hydrophobic (and lipophilic) LAs have higher potency. Lipophilic compounds more readily cross nerve cell membranes and bind more avidly to their hydrophobic effect site. Other factors such as nerve fiber size, myelination, pH, frequency of nerve firing, and plasma electrolyte also impact potency.

Speed of LA onset is affected by the pKa of a drug, as well as factors like lipid solubility and LA concentration. The pKa of an LA can be defined as the pH level at which the LA molecule is found in equal ionized and non-ionized concentrations. LAs are weak bases. The closer a specific LA's pKa is to physiologic pH, the more non-ionized form exists and the more readily it crosses nerve cell membrane, resulting in faster block onset [3]. Thus, adding alkaline sodium bicarbonate ($NaHCO_3$) to lidocaine will speed onset of conduction blockade by increasing tissue pH. Unfortunately, $NaHCO_3$ will cause drug precipitation with ropivacaine and bupivacaine, so it should not be used with them [4]. 2-Chloroprocaine is an exception to the rule of pKa determining LA onset. Despite its high pKa, it has a fast onset, due to its high concentration (3%) [1].

Duration of LA effect is related to the degree of protein binding. LAs bind plasma alpha-1-glycoprotein and, to a lesser extent, albumin. Protein binding will increase block duration by slowing drug elimination. Lipophilic LAs are also more slowly cleared. Liposome-encapsulated drug formulations (liposomal bupivacaine) have been developed to provide sustained release of LA with prolonged duration.

Anyone administering an LA should know its maximum safe dose and be aware of the risk of LAST (Table 31.1). The site of administration (Table 31.2) and use of vasoconstrictors (e.g., epinephrine) effect the rate of systemic absorption which in turn increases time to peak drug plasma levels and risk of LAST with high doses or inadvertent intravenous (IV) administration. Vasoconstrictors like epinephrine slow

Table 31.2 Rate of local anesthetic absorption by route administered

Intravenous > Tracheal > Intercostal > Caudal > Paracervical > Epidural > Brachial Plexus > Spinal > Subcutaneous

Table 31.3 Commonly used local anesthetic concentrations

Local anesthetic	Analgesic concentrations	Anesthetic concentrations
Bupivacaine	0.1%, 0.125%	**0.25%, 0.5%, 0.75%**
Ropivacaine	**0.2%**, 0.25%,	**0.5%, 1%**
Lidocaine	0.5%, **1%**	**1.5%, 2%**
Mepivacaine	1%	**1.5%, 2%**
2-Chloroprocaine	1%	2%, **3%**

Bolded concentrations are commercially available formulations. Other concentrations are made by dilution

Table 31.4 Peripheral nerve block local anesthetics [2]

Local anesthetic	Onset	Duration (min)	Duration with added epinephrine (min)	Maximum recommended LA dose
Bupivacaine	Slow	480–780	600–900	2.5 mg/kg (200 mg max)
Ropivacaine	Slow	360–480	480–600	2.5 mg/kg (225 mg max)
Lidocaine	Rapid	90–120	120–180	5 mg/kg (300 mg max)
Mepivacaine	Rapid	100–150	120–220	5 mg/kg (400 mg max)

uptake and prolong duration of lidocaine, mepivacaine, and chloroprocaine, though there is little effect on ropivacaine or bupivacaine.

Why Use Local Anesthetic Regional Techniques for the Chronic Non-cancer Patient With Acute Pain?

Regional anesthesia using LAs and adjuncts avoids patient tolerance to opioids or other medications, and when performed correctly, is highly effective. Opioid dose escalation can be avoided and the risk of a transition from acute to chronic pain may be decreased, with the best data around the use of neuraxial techniques.

Multiple formulations of each local anesthetic are commercially available. The specific drug and formulation chosen should be based on desired density of blockade (analgesic vs. anesthetic block), intended duration, and speed of onset. Higher concentrations of LAs are can produce profound, surgical anesthetic block, while lower concentrations can be used for analgesia (Table 31.3).

Characteristics of the depth and duration of conduction blockade vary significantly by the site administered, even when using the same medication. Tables 31.4, 31.5, and 31.6 show characteristics of peripheral nerve, epidural, and spinal blockade, respectively. A common theme is that bupivacaine and ropivacaine have a longer onset and duration than shorter acting LAs such as lidocaine, mepivacaine, and especially chloroprocaine. Table 31.7 shows alternative routes of local anesthetics for acute pain.

Table 31.5 Epidural local anesthetics [2]

Local anesthetic	Onset	Duration (min)	Duration with added Epinephrine (min)
Bupivacaine	Slow	165–225	180–240
Chloroprocaine	Fast	45–60	60–90
Lidocaine	Fast	80–120	120–180
Mepivacaine	Fast	90–140	140–200
Ropivacaine	Slow	140–200	160–220

Table 31.6 Spinal (Subarachnoid) local anesthetics [2]

Local anesthetic	Onset (min)	Duration (min)	Commonly used dose (mg)	Time to ambulation (min)
Bupivacaine	4–8	130–230	5–15	160–310
Ropivacaine	3–8	80–210	12–18	160–305
Mepivacaine	2–4	120–180	40–60	145–240
Lidocaine	3–5	60–150	30–80	100–185
Chloroprocaine	2–4	40–90	40–60	85–185

Table 31.7 Alternative routes of local anesthetics for acute pain [5]

Route	Commonly used dose
Intravenous Lidocaine	0.5–2 mg/min
Transdermal Lidocaine	4% or 5% patch
Tumescent Lidocaine	Maximum 45 mg/kg with liposuction
Oral Mexiletine	150–250 mg PO TID

Why Use Intravenous Lidocaine for the Chronic Non-cancer Patient with Acute Pain?

Lidocaine intravenous (IV) infusions have been used in multiple contexts, including as therapy for hyperalgesia and neuropathic pain. The best evidence of benefit comes in abdominal surgery, where prolonged infusions of lidocaine result in decreased pain, lower opioid use, and faster return of bowel function [4]. This is thought to result from effects on multiple pathways, including sodium channels and separate anti-inflammatory effects.

What Are the Risks of Local Anesthetic Administration?

The risks of administering local anesthetics are numerous, but broadly fall into risks related to the effects of the medications and where they are administered or those due to the block placement or performance (Table 31.8). Permanent or prolonged nerve injury has an incidence of 2–4 per 10,000 blocks.

Table 31.8 Risks of nerve block [6]

Related to medication or injection site	Related to block placement
Local Anesthetic Systemic Toxicity	Block failure
Transient Neurologic Symptoms (TNS)	Nerve injury
Falls	Bleeding
Urinary retention	Infection or abscess
Phrenic blockade (shortness of breath)	Post-dural puncture headache
Hypotension	Pneumothorax
Epidural or Intrathecal spread (high block)	

Table 31.9 Variable presentation of LAST: signs and symptoms [2]

Neurologic	Seizure, agitation, loss of consciousness, dizziness, tinnitus, perioral numbness, drowsiness, dysarthria, dysphoria, confusion
Cardiovascular	Bradycardia, asystole, tachycardia, hypotension, wide complex rhythm, ventricular ectopy, st changes, chest pain, dyspnea, hypertension, ventricular tachycardia or fibrillation

Table 31.10 Local anesthetic systemic toxicity prevention [2]

Decrease LA volume administered
Minimize LA concentration
Aspirate before administering LA
Inject in small increments
Use epinephrine to allow recognition of IV injection
Use ultrasound guidance

Local Anesthetic Systemic Toxicity

Local anesthetic systemic toxicity (LAST) is a life-threatening complication of local anesthetic administration regardless of the route it is given. Signs and symptoms fall into the category of neurologic or cardiovascular effects (Table 31.9). The presentation can be highly variable and the presence of any signs or symptoms around the time of LA administration should be carefully considered as potential initial presentation of LAST. Cardiac signs and symptoms may be the initial presenting sign of LAST in a patient under general anesthesia. Prevention of LAST is also critical (Table 31.10).

Therapy for LAST differs from ACLS in a number of ways. Vasopressin, calcium channel blockers, local anesthetics, and propofol should be avoided in LAST treatment. Epinephrine dosing should be reduced to ≤1 mcg/kg. Lipid emulsion therapy should be initiated, and the cardiac bypass team alerted for potential bypass initiation in refractory LAST (Tables 31.11 and 31.12).

Table 31.11 What to do when LAST is suspected [2]	Stop injection of local anesthetic Call for help, alert cardiac bypass team Initiate lipid emulsion therapy (Table 31.12) Control seizures (give benzodiazepine) Manage airway—ventilate with $FiO_2 = 1$ Initiate good, high quality ACLS with slight differences Monitor for 4–6 h after return of spontaneous circulation

Table 31.12 Lipid emulsion therapy [2]	Bolus dose 1.5 mL/kg lipid emulsion (20%) Infuse 0.25 mL/kg/min lipid emulsion May repeat bolus May double infusion rate Max 10 mL/kg intralipid

References

1. Spinal E, Blocks C. Maternal and fetal physiology and anesthesia. In: Butterworth IV JF, Mackey DC, Wasnick JD, editors. Morgan & Mikhail's clinical anesthesiology. 5th ed. New York, NY: McGraw-Hill; 2013.
2. Miller RD. Miller's anesthesia. 8th ed. Philadelphia, PA: Elsevier/Saunders; 2015.
3. Williams DJ, Walker JD. A nomogram for calculating the maximum dose of local anaesthetic. Anaesthesia. 2014;69(8):847–53.
4. Neal JM, Mulroy MF, Weinberg GL. American society of regional anesthesia and pain medicine checklist for managing local anesthetic systemic toxicity: 2012 version. Reg Anesth Pain Med. 2012;37(1):16–8.
5. Sun Y, Li T, Wang N, Yun Y, Gan TJ. Perioperative systemic lidocaine for postoperative analgesia and recovery after abdominal surgery. Dis Colon Rectum. 2012;55(11):1183–94.
6. Horlocker TT. Complications of regional anesthesia and acute pain management. Anesthesiol Clin. 2011;29(2):257–78.

NMDA Antagonists

32

Michael Kent and David A. Edwards

Introduction

Ketamine, a phenylpiperidine derivative, produces a strong analgesic effect through inhibition of the N-methyl-D-aspartate receptor as well as through other systems such as mu, muscarinic, and monoaminergic receptors [1]. Numerous trials have established the analgesic and opioid sparing qualities of ketamine in acute, chronic, and acute on chronic pain states [2, 3]. Specifically, ketamine is particularly used for pain in the setting of opioid tolerance, neuropathic pain, pain unrelieved by opioids, severe acute pain, and states involving central sensitization. While ketamine has demonstrated a preventative effect in the acute setting and a lasting benefit in the chronic pain setting, these results still warrant further investigation and classification [2, 3]. With a notable safety record when administered in subanesthetic doses, ketamine should be considered early in the treatment of pain in hospitalized patients with pre-existing pain conditions.

Routes

While ketamine can be administered via numerous routes (IM/IV/PO/PR/TD), intravenous administration is the most common. Subanesthetic (low dose) dosing is often considered to be less than 1.2 mg/kg/h and <1 mg/kg for bolus dosing [4]. However, practical low dose ketamine infusions often range between 0.1–0.3 mg/kg/h.

M. Kent
Department of Anesthesiology, Duke University Health System, Durham, NC, USA

D. A. Edwards (✉)
Departments of Anesthesiology and Neurological Surgery, Vanderbilt University Medical Center, Nashville, TN, USA
e-mail: david.a.edwards@vumc.org

© Springer Nature Switzerland AG 2022
D. A. Edwards et al. (eds.), *Hospitalized Chronic Pain Patient*,
https://doi.org/10.1007/978-3-031-08376-1_32

Table 32.1 Common routes and dosing for inpatient ketamine use [5]

Route	Dose	Bioavailability (%)	Comments
PO	0.5 mg/kg (racemic mixture) q6–8	20	• Decreased side effects compared to IV administration • Compounding often required
IV Infusion (low dose)	0.06–0.2 mg/kg/h	90	• Suggest starting lower in elderly population • Bolus PCA function may be added (1–5 mg q 30 min)
IV Bolus	0.25–0.5 mg/kg	90	• Typically used for breakthrough or acute pain. May increase psychomimetic side effects with rapid administration. Consider smaller loading doses 5–10 mg prior to infusion

While intranasal and transdermal are available, their applicability to the inpatient setting is limited

Table 32.2 Ketamine pharmacology [1]

Metabolism	Cytochrome p450 dependent (CYP3A4, CYP2B6, CYP2C9), Primary metabolite: Norketamine
Renal dosing	No dose adjustment required. However, vigilance required with accompanying comorbidities
Half life	Elimination half-life → 2–3 h

In general, no additional monitoring is required during ketamine infusions. Please see Tables 32.1 and 32.2 for commonly used routes/dosing and salient pharmacology.

Side Effects/Toxicity

Ketamine has long carried a concern for significant side effects particularly focused on psychomimetic symptoms (Table 32.3). Within low dose regimens, these side effects are negligibly increased compared to placebo [3]. In general, no monitoring is required during ketamine infusions. Further, if symptoms are due to ketamine, return to baseline can be expected within 15–30 min following cessation of infusion. Hepatotoxicity has been documented in repeat ketamine infusions in small series. Ketamine induced cystitis has also been observed in chronic recreational users of ketamine [7].

Conclusion

Ketamine administration should be considered for hospitalized patients with chronic pain if common modalities do not provide sufficient analgesia. Low dose ketamine infusion has displayed clear benefits in acute, acute on chronic, and chronic pain states. Education and engagement of ancillary staff (e.g., nursing, pharmacy, etc.) is critical to effective treatment protocols.

Table 32.3 Ketamine side effects [6]

Psychomimetic	• Minimal increase in hallucinations/vivid dreams/blurry vision compared to placebo
	• Rapid resolution with decrease in dose or discontinuation
	• Dose dependent relationship
	• Co-administration of clonidine 0.1–0.2 mg qD or low dose PRN benzodiazepine can be used to mitigate side effects
Intracranial dynamics	• No increase in intracranial pressure in traumatic/non-traumatic neurologic conditions
Sedation	• Dose dependent and reversed with decrease in dose or cessation of infusion
Nausea/Vomiting	• Minimal impact with low dose infusion
	• May be present with prolonged high dose infusions
Cardiovascular Stimulation	• Unlikely with low dose administration
	• Consider telemetry for patient with significant cardiovascular comorbidities
Cognitive	• Unclear impact for chronic therapeutic administration. Recent small series suggest deficits in executive functioning

References

1. Vadivelu N, Schermer E, Kodumudi V, Belani K, Urman RD, Kaye AD. Role of ketamine for analgesia in adults and children. J Anaesthesiol Clin Pharmacol. 2016;32(3):298–306.
2. Niesters M, Martini C, Dahan A. Ketamine for chronic pain: risks and benefits. Br J Clin Pharmacol. 2014;77(2):357–67.
3. Jouguelet Lacoste J, La Colla L, Schilling D, Chelly JE. The use of intravenous infusion or single dose of low-dose ketamine for postoperative analgesia: a review of the current literature. Pain Med. 2015;16(2):383–403.
4. Schmid RL, Sandler AN, Katz J. Use and efficacy of low-dose ketamine in the management of acute postoperative pain: a review of current techniques and outcomes. Pain. 1999;82(2):111–25.
5. Blonk MI, Koder BG, van den Bemt PMLA, Huygen FJPM. Use of oral ketamine in chronic pain management: a review. Eur J Pain. 2010;14(5):466–72.
6. Kim M, Cho S, Lee J-H. the effects of long-term ketamine treatment on cognitive function in complex regional pain syndrome: a preliminary study. Pain Med. 2016;17(8):1447–51.
7. Jhang JF, Hsu YH, Kuo HC. Possible pathophysiology of ketamine-related cystitis and associated treatment strategies. Int J Urol. 2015;22(9):816–25.

Alpha-2 Agonists

33

Benjamin J. MacDougall and Puneet Mishra

What Are Alpha-2 Agonists?

Within the adrenergic signalling system, norepinephrine and epinephrine act as ligands on alpha and beta receptors. The alpha subtype of receptors is further subdivided into α1 and α2. The former are primarily post-junctional, while the latter are primarily pre-junctional. They exert differing effects via second messenger.

Alpha-2 receptors are found throughout the central and peripheral nervous system, and their agonists are increasingly used in the treatment of both acute and chronic pain. There are three further subtypes of the α2 receptor, known as α2A, α2B, and α2C. Alpha-2A and -2C are located in the central nervous system, while -2B are more commonly on vascular smooth muscle.

Regardless of the subtype, receptor activation results in inhibition of adenylyl cyclase and therefore decreased cyclic adenosine monophosphate (cAMP) production. This decrease in cAMP production has numerous downstream effects, with the overall effect depending on the location and type of the receptor. With α2A activation, the clinically important downstream effects include inhibition of N-type voltage sensitive calcium channels, resulting in decreased presynaptic norepinephrine release, as well as activation of potassium channels, causing neuronal hyperpolarization and attenuated neural transmission [1]. With α2B activation, the important downstream effects include vascular smooth muscle contraction.

Alpha-2 agonists exert anti-nociceptive action by both central and peripheral pathways, some of which remain to be fully elucidated. With regard to the central pathway, there are α2 receptors in the dorsal horn of the spinal cord as well as in the locus coeruleus. Stimulating α2 receptors in the dorsal horn results in reduced release of substance P and inhibits nociceptive neural pathways. Activity in the

B. J. MacDougall · P. Mishra (✉)
Department of Anesthesiology, Vanderbilt University Medical Center, Nashville, TN, USA
e-mail: benjamin.macdougall@vumc.org; puneet.mishra@vumc.org

© Springer Nature Switzerland AG 2022
D. A. Edwards et al. (eds.), *Hospitalized Chronic Pain Patient*,
https://doi.org/10.1007/978-3-031-08376-1_33

locus coeruleus results in sedation as well as inhibition of the sympathetic stress response. Peripheral mechanisms are not well-understood, but it has been proposed that they may cause dose-related inhibition of C-fibers and A-α fibers [2].

Clonidine

Clonidine is an α2 agonist with an α2 to α1 specificity of 200:1. Its anti-nociceptive properties have been well-studied, particularly in the perioperative setting, where it has been administered via oral, intravenous, transdermal, local infiltration, epidural, intrathecal, perineural, and intra-articular routes.

A 2012 meta-analysis demonstrated statistically significant decrease in morphine equivalent administration at 12 and 24 h postoperatively when clonidine IV (doses ranging from 2–5 μg/kg bolus with 0.3–0.5 μg/kg/h) or PO (doses from 2 to 3 μg/kg or 150–300 μg) was administered. This effect is attributed to clonidine's ability to cross the blood brain barrier, where CSF concentrations are noted to be approximately 50% of plasma concentrations [3].

The benefits of clonidine when administered perineurally as an adjunct to local anesthetics for nerve blocks have been well-documented. Duration of analgesia was uniformly increased with use of clonidine, regardless of the block location or the type of local anesthetic used, though this effect was seen less consistently for long-acting local anesthetics. Clonidine has also been used intrathecally both alone and as an adjunct to local anesthetic. In both circumstances, pain scores were lower and time to first supplementary analgesic was increased [4, 5]. Epidural administration of clonidine has also been extensively studied, but the study designs and protocols are quite varied, so it has been difficult to draw definitive conclusions about efficacy. However, individual studies have suggested a positive analgesic effect when the medication was administered epidurally [2].

In addition to its anti-nociceptive properties, clonidine is also used as an antihypertensive, in the treatment of perioperative anxiety, and to alleviate the sympathetic effects of numerous withdrawal syndromes (including opioids, alcohol, benzodiazepines, nicotine). Furthermore, it can be used to treat attention deficit hyperactivity disorder (ADHD; mechanism of this described below under guanfacine). Like tizanidine (described below), it also has some use in treating spasticity.

Metabolism

Clonidine is metabolized by the liver into inactive metabolites, and a large proportion is excreted unchanged by the kidney. Accordingly, half life can be significantly prolonged in patients with renal dysfunction. The most common adverse effects are hypotension, dizziness, somnolence, and fatigue, which are easily understood given the drug's mechanism. Should the medication be stopped suddenly, significant rebound hypertension is possible, so tapering is recommended [1].

Tizanidine

Tizanidine is a central α2 agonist FDA-approved for the management of spasticity, and commonly used in clinical practice for the treatment of muscle spasms and/or musculoskeletal pain. It is administered orally, and exerts its antispastic effect via presynaptic inhibition of spinal interneurons and motor neurons.

The role of tizanidine is best established in the treatment of spasticity secondary to neurologic injury (e.g., stroke, spinal cord injury) or disease (e.g., multiple sclerosis, amyotrophic lateral sclerosis). A number of studies have confirmed tizanidine is superior to placebo and equally effective compared to diazepam or baclofen in controlling symptoms of spasticity [6, 7].

In patients undergoing general endotracheal anesthesia, oral premedication with tizanidine attenuates the hypertensive response during laryngoscopy, reduces the required maintenance dose of anesthetic, and prolongs spinal anesthesia [8–11]. In the acute postoperative setting, tizanidine has been shown to decrease pain scores, decrease analgesic consumption, and hasten return to normal activity [12, 13].

Tizanidine has demonstrated efficacy in the treatment of neuropathic pain [14], myofascial pain [15, 16], and acute low back pain [17]. Furthermore, in addition to its antinociceptive effects, it has also been shown to exhibit gastroprotective effects when combined with NSAIDs [18].

Metabolism

Tizanidine undergoes significant first pass hepatic metabolism to inactive metabolites excreted through urine and feces [19]. Thus, it should be avoided in hepatic impairment and used with caution in renal impairment. The most common adverse effect is sedation (48–92%), necessitating caution in patients taking concurrent CNS depressants. Hypotension is the second most common (16–33%) adverse effect. In patients receiving moderate to high doses (e.g., >10 mg/day) for extended periods (e.g. >9 weeks), tizanidine should be tapered gradually to avoid rebound symptoms of hypertension, tachycardia, and hypertonia.

Dexmedetomidine

Dexmedetomidine is a potent α2 agonist medication, with an estimated α2 to α1 specificity of 1620:1. It can be administered via intravenous, buccal, intranasal, intramuscular, intra-articular, perineural, intrathecal, or epidural routes. The primary clinical use of dexmedetomidine capitalizes upon its sedative and hypnotic effects, which are exerted in the locus coeruleus. It is used as a primary or adjunct sedative medication in both an intensive care and procedural setting, and it is also used for prevention and treatment of emergence delirium.

The use of dexmedetomidine as an anti-nociceptive agent occurs primarily in the perioperative setting. When used intraoperatively as an infusion (0.1–1 μg/kg/h as a bolus or continued throughout the anesthetic), meta-analyses have demonstrated statistically significant decreases in morphine requirements at 2, 12, and 24 h as well as significant decrease in VAS pain scores at 1 and 24 h post-operatively. There have been no reports that investigate the effect of perioperative dexmedetomidine on chronic pain or hyperalgesia on a longer time scale [3].

There have been a number of small studies using intrathecal, epidural, and caudal dexmedetomidine in addition to local anesthetic that demonstrated superior intraoperative and post-operative analgesia compared to local anesthetic alone or local anesthetic with clonidine. Similar improvements in sensory blockade have been noted when using dexmedetomidine with local anesthetic in peripheral nerve blocks. Of note, there is also evidence that IV dexmedetomidine is associated with prolonged block duration with spinal anesthesia and reduced opioid requirements following shoulder surgery under interscalene block [2].

The sympatholytic action of dexmedetomidine can result in hypotension and bradycardia and is the primary reason for discontinuation. This effect can be seen not only with intravenous administration but also with perineural and neuraxial administration. Conversely, when administered via rapid bolus administration, dexmedetomidine can induce hypertension via stimulation of peripheral α2B receptors, which causes vascular smooth muscle constriction. This latter effect is rarely relevant clinically.

Metabolism

Dexmedetomidine is metabolized hepatically and primarily renally excreted; there are no known active metabolites.

Guanfacine

Guanfacine is an oral α2 agonist with more limited use in pain management but with a role in treating opioid withdrawal and behavioral disorders. It is currently being studied to determine whether or not it may have a role in preventing opioid induced hyperalgesia and tolerance.

It is highly selective for the α2A receptor subtype, which is found centrally. This leads to a centrally mediated sympatholytic effect profile, decreasing heart rate and blood pressure, which accounts for the drug's use as an antihypertensive agent. It is also used in this capacity as an adjunct for patients undergoing opioid withdrawal; compared with clonidine, it may be more effective while causing less hypotension [20]. There are also post-synaptic α2A receptors in the prefrontal cortex, and binding of the drug to these receptors causes improved neural connectivity in this region of the brain, improving working memory and behavioral inhibition [21, 22]. These effects are the basis for its use as a medication for ADHD and for other disorders of the prefrontal cortex.

Table 33.1 Summary of alpha-agonists

	Route of administration	Metabolism/ excretion	Half life	Clinical pitfalls
Clonidine	IV, oral, perineural, intrathecal, epidural, transdermal	M: Liver (50%) E: 40–60% unchanged in urine, 20% bile/feces	12–16 h	Rebound HTN with sudden cessation
Tizanidine	Oral	M: Liver E: 60% urine, 20% feces	2.5 h	Sedation, hypotension, rebound HTN, tachycardia, hypertonia w sudden cessation
Dexmedetomidine	IV, oral, perineural, intrathecal, epidural, intranasal	M: Liver E: 95% urine, 4% feces	2 h; context-sensitive halftime increase w/infusion duration	Hypotension, bradycardia
Guanfacine	Oral	M: Liver (50%) E: 50% urine	17 h (for both IR and ER)	Drowsiness, dizziness, GI distress

IV intravenous, *HTN* hypertension, *IR* immediate release, *ER* extended release

Metabolism

Guanfacine is metabolized hepatically and renally excreted. The half life of the immediate release formulation is approximately 17 hours but can range from 10–30 h; the extended-release half life is similar. The formulations differ in their time to peak effect, which is 2.6 h for the immediate release and 4 to 8 h for the extended release. Adverse effects cited with use of this medication include drowsiness, dizziness, and fatigue, which are predictable given the drug's mechanism of action. Mood and gastrointestinal side effects are also common. Cardiovascular side effects are less common with this α2 agent than others in this class, though they are possible. Table 33.1 below provides a summary of alpha-agonists that are commonly prescribed.

References

1. Giovannitti JA Jr, Thoms SM, Crawford JJ. Alpha-2 adrenergic receptor agonists: a review of current clinical applications. Anesth Prog. 2015;62(1):31–9.
2. Chan AK, Cheung CW, Chong YK. Alpha-2 agonists in acute pain management. Expert Opin Pharmacother. 2010;11(17):2849–68.
3. Blaudszun G, Lysakowski C, Elia N, Tramèr MR. Effect of perioperative systemic α2 agonists on postoperative morphine consumption and pain intensity: systematic review and meta-analysis of randomized controlled trials. Anesthesiology. 2012;116(6):1312–22.

4. Filos KS, Goudas LC, Patroni O, Polyzou V. Hemodynamic and analgesic profile after intrathecal clonidine in humans. A dose-response study. Anesthesiology. 1994;81:591–601. Discussion 27A–28A
5. Elia N, Culebras X, Mazza C, et al. Clonidine as an adjuvant to intrathecal local anesthetics for surgery: systematic review of randomized trials. Reg Anesth Pain Med. 2008;33(2):159–67.
6. Smith C, Birnbaum G, Carter JL. Tizanidine treatment of spasticity caused by multiple sclerosis: results of a double-blind, placebo-controlled trial. US Tizanidine Study Group. Neurology. 1994;44:S34–42.
7. Wagstaff AJ, Bryson HM. Tizanidine: a review of its pharmacology, clinical efficacy and tolerability in the management of spasticity associated with cerebral and spinal disorders. Drugs. 1997;53:435–52.
8. Tabari M, Alipour M, Esalati H. Evaluation of oral tizanidine effects on intra operative hemodynamic responses during direct laryngoscopy under general anesthesia. Iran Red Crescent Med J. 2013;15:541–6.
9. Takenaka M, Iida H, Kasamatsu M, et al. Tizanidine for preanesthetic medication. Masui. 1996;45:971–5.
10. Wajima Z, Yoshikawa T, Ogura A, et al. Oral tizanidine, an alpha2-adrenoceptor agonist, reduces the minimum alveolar concentration of sevoflurane in human adults. Anesth Analg. 2002;95:393–6.
11. Omote K, Satoh O, Sonoda H, et al. Effects of oral alpha 2 adrenergic agonists, clonidine and tizanidine, on tetracaine spinal anesthesia. Masui. 1995;44:816–23.
12. Yazicioğlu D, Caparlar C, Akkaya T, Mercan U, Kulaçoğlu H. Tizanidine for the management of acute postoperative pain after inguinal hernia repair. Eur J Anaesthesiol. 2016;33(3):215–22.
13. Talakoub R, Abbasi S, Maghami E, Zavareh SM. The effect of oral tizanidine on postoperative pain relief after elective laparoscopic cholecystectomy. Adv Biomed Res. 2016;5:19.
14. Semenchuk MR, Sherman S. Effectiveness of tizanidine in neuropathic pain: an open-label study. J Pain. 2000;1(4):285–92.
15. Malanga GA, Gwynn MW, Smith R, Miller D. Tizanidine is effective in the treatment of myofascial pain syndrome. Pain Physician. 2002;5(4):422–32.
16. Manfredini D, Romagnoli M, Cantini E, Bosco M. Efficacy of tizanidine hydrochloride in the treatment of myofascial face pain. Minerva Med. 2004;95(2):165–7.
17. Berry H, Hutchinson DR. A multicentre placebo-controlled study in general practice to evaluate the efficacy and safety of tizanidine in acute low-back pain. J Int Med Res. 1988;16(2):75–82. https://doi.org/10.1177/030006058801600201.
18. Sirdalud Ternelin Asia-Pacific Study Group. Efficacy and gastroprotective effects of tizanidine plus diclofenac versus placebo plus diclofenac in patients with painful muscle spasms. Curr Ther Res. 1998;59:13–22.
19. Ghanavatian S, Derian A. Tizanidine. [Updated 2020 Aug 11]. In: StatPearls [Internet]. Treasure Island, FL: StatPearls Publishing; 2020. Available from: https://www.ncbi.nlm.nih.gov/books/NBK519505/
20. San L, Camí J, Peri JM, Mata R, Porta M. Efficacy of clonidine, guanfacine and methadone in the rapid detoxification of heroin addicts: a controlled clinical trial. Br J Addict. 1990;85(1):141–7.
21. Arnsten AF. The use of α2A adrenergic agonists for the treatment of attention-deficit/hyperactivity disorder. Expert Rev Neurother. 2010;10(10):1595–605.
22. Wang M, et al. Alpha2A-adrenoceptors strengthen working memory networks by inhibiting cAMP-HCN channel signaling in prefrontal cortex. Cell. 2007;129(2):397–410.

Gabapentin and Pregabalin

34

Christopher M. Sobey and David Byrne

Basics

The gabapentinoids, gabapentin and pregabalin, are gamma-aminobutyric acid (GABA) analogues that are currently approved for post-herpetic neuralgia and as an adjunct for epilepsy. Pregabalin is additionally approved for the treatment of fibromyalgia and neuropathic pain associated with diabetes mellitus or spinal cord injury. Both are often used off label due to their favorable therapeutic indices for a variety of pain syndromes, especially those involving neuropathic pain.

Mechanism of Action

While the gabapentinoids were originally developed as GABA analogues with anti-spasmodic and antiepileptic characteristics, their antinociceptive qualities were found serendipitously. Despite their similarities to GABA, they likely exert a negligible effect on GABA receptors. Their main mechanism of action involves selective inhibitory effect on voltage-gated calcium channels containing the $\alpha_2\delta$ subunit. Presynaptic calcium influx modulation likely attenuates glutamate release in the nociceptive pathways, thus reducing pain transmission, hyperalgesia, and central sensitization [1].

Administered orally, gabapentin and pregabalin are absorbed both by diffusion and by the carrier-mediated amino acid transport system. Gabapentin transport is limited to the duodenum resulting in a saturable transport system that leads to an inverse relationship between dose and bioavailability. This ceiling effect may

C. M. Sobey (✉)
Department of Anesthesiology, Vanderbilt University Medical Center, Nashville, TN, USA
e-mail: christopher.m.sobey@vumc.org

D. Byrne
U.S. Anesthesia Partners, Dallas, TX, USA

© Springer Nature Switzerland AG 2022
D. A. Edwards et al. (eds.), *Hospitalized Chronic Pain Patient*,
https://doi.org/10.1007/978-3-031-08376-1_34

explain why dose escalations at higher doses produce limited benefit and side effects. Pregabalin, however, is absorbed throughout the small intestine and demonstrates more linear pharmacokinetics [2, 3]. Gabapentin is not metabolized, but is eliminated unchanged solely by renal clearance. Plasma clearance is directly proportional to creatinine clearance. The elimination half-life ranges of gabapentin and pregabalin are 4.8–8.7 h and 5.5–6.3 h, respectively [4].

Dosing

Dosing for inpatients with normal renal function usually starts at 300 mg q8h and can be titrated up incrementally as benefit and side effects allow. The maximum daily dose is 3600 mg total daily in divided doses, however there is generally limited benefit in increasing the total daily dose over 1800 mg. Since elimination is dependent on renal clearance, the calculated creatinine clearance must be monitored in patients receiving gabapentin and pregabalin [5–7]. Supplemental dosing of 100–300 mg after dialysis may be reasonable since these medications are cleared with hemodialysis. Differences between pregabalin and gabapentin are modest at best in postoperative pain scores and opioid consumption, however cost may be an important consideration for some patients as pregabalin is still patent protected while gabapentin is available as a generic [8]. Table 34.1 shows the dose correction for both pregabalin and gabapentin in patients with impaired kidney function.

Adverse Effects

Side effects are usually mild but can be dose limiting and affect patient satisfaction. The most common side effects are sedation, lightheadedness, visual changes, confusion, and dizziness [3, 5, 8]. Peripheral edema is also a known side effect. These are more likely in the elderly and at increased doses. In toxic levels seen in patients with changes in renal function or intentional/accidental overdose, coma and respiratory depression can result. The gabapentinoids can be removed by renal replacement therapies. Unfortunately, the assay for serum gabapentin levels is not available in most labs.

A major complication that can develop with high-dose gabapentin and pregabalin use is the risk for withdrawal. Almost all reported gabapentin withdrawal case reports occurred after abrupt discontinuation of high-dose gabapentin, but

Table 34.1 Pregabalin and gabapentin dosing in renal dysfunction [8]

Creatinine clearance, ml/min	Maximal daily pregabalin dose (mg)	Maximal daily gabapentin dose (mg)
>60	600	3600
30–60	300	1400
15–30	150	700
15	75	300

withdrawal after taper has also been reported [9]. The clinical presentation of gabapentin withdrawal appears to be similar to that of benzodiazepines: seizure, agitation and anxiety, diaphoresis, somatic pain, confusion, tremulousness, gastrointestinal distress, and autonomic instability [8, 9]. Various tapering schedules have been successful but should likely be done in over at least a week on patients taking more than 900 mg daily of gabapentin. Some recommend a similar taper schedule to benzodiazepines occurring over weeks. Patients taking less than 900 mg daily may not need to be tapered.

Gabapentin and pregabalin are Pregnancy category C. Some studies have shown developmental abnormalities in animals exposed to clinical doses of these medications during gestation. Although the literature is sparse, gabapentinoids should be used during pregnancy only if the potential benefit justifies the potential risk to the fetus.

References

1. Sills GJ. The mechanisms of action of gabapentin and pregabalin. Curr Opin Pharmacol. 2006;6(1):108–13.
2. Piyapolrungroj N, Li C, Bockbrader H, Liu G, Fleisher D. Mucosal uptake of gabapentin (neurontin) vs. pregabalin in the small intestine. Pharm Res. 2001;18:1126–30.
3. Chang CY, Challa CK, Shah J, Eloy JD. Gabapentin in acute postoperative pain management. Biomed Res Int. 2014;2014:631756.
4. Weinbroum AA. Non-opioid IV adjuvants in the perioperative period: pharmacological and clinical aspects of ketamine and gabapentinoids. Pharmacol Res. 2012;65:411–29.
5. Miller A, Price G. Gabapentin toxicity in renal failure: the importance of dose adjustment. Pain Med. 2009;10(1):190–2.
6. Pregabalin [package insert]. New York Parke-Davis, a Division of Pfizer; 2009.
7. Gabapentin [package insert]. New York Parke-Davis, a Division of Pfizer; 2012.
8. Schmidt PC, Ruchelli G, Mackey SC, Carroll IR. Perioperative gabapentinoids: choice of agent, dose, timing, and effects on chronic postsurgical pain. Anesthesiology. 2013;119(5):1215–21.
9. Mah L, Hart M. Gabapentin withdrawal: case report in an older adult and review of the literature. J Am Geriatr Soc. 2013;61(9):1635–7.

Tricyclic Antidepressants and Serotonin-Norepinephrine Reuptake Inhibitors

35

Shaun Kuoni, Maxwell James, and Christopher M. Sobey

Tricyclic Antidepressants

Tricyclic antidepressants (TCAs) are a group of compounds comprised of both secondary and tertiary amines that were initially introduced for treatment of depression in the 1950s. Since that time, TCAs have been shown to be beneficial in number of chronic neuropathic pain conditions including diabetic neuropathy, trigeminal neuralgia, post-herpetic neuralgia, and central post-stroke pain [1]. They act primarily by inhibiting presynaptic reuptake of both serotonin and norepinephrine which results in inhibition of central and ascending pain pathways in the dorsal horn. In addition to their effect on serotonin and norepinephrine, TCAs have been shown to be particularly effective in neuropathic pain secondary to blockade of central alpha-adrenergic receptors, NMDA receptors on second order neurons, sodium channels on both central and peripheral nerves, and calcium channels [1]. Common TCAs in use today include amitriptyline, imipramine, clomipramine, nortriptyline, and desipramine.

Initiation and Side Effects

Outpatient initiation of these medications for both chronic pain or depression is ideal for a variety of reasons, and the inpatient setting poses many challenges to effective initiation and titration of TCAs. TCAs, like many other classes of antidepressants, take anywhere from 1–6 weeks for onset of clinically significant effect. It

S. Kuoni
The NeuroMedical Center Clinic, Hammond, LA, USA

M. James (✉) · C. M. Sobey
Department of Anesthesiology, Vanderbilt University Medical Center, Nashville, TN, USA
e-mail: maxwell.b.james@vumc.org; christopher.m.sobey@vumc.org

© Springer Nature Switzerland AG 2022
D. A. Edwards et al. (eds.), *Hospitalized Chronic Pain Patient*,
https://doi.org/10.1007/978-3-031-08376-1_35

is believed that this delay in effect is primarily because these medications work through the neuroplasticity to alter gene transcription and subsequently neurotransmitter and receptor expression [2]. Additionally, TCAs are metabolized by the CYP2D6 enzymatic system, and population wide genetic polymorphism in CYP2D6 can result in a wide range of therapeutic and toxic doses that can make initial dose finding difficult [1]. For this reason, TCAs should be initiated in a setting where doses can be carefully titrated, and side effects monitored for over a period of weeks to months until therapeutic dosing is confirmed.

Further complicating this is the fact that TCAs have the potential for interactions with several medications that are common to the chronic pain population. The SSRIs fluoxetine and paroxetine are potent inhibitors of CYP2D6, and any variability in administration or dosing for patients maintained on these medications could result in serotonin toxicity or ineffectiveness if TCAs are initiated during that same time [1]. Additionally, the serotonergic action of tramadol leads to the potential for serotonin syndrome when tramadol is co-administered with a TCA. While it is not contraindicated, care should be taken when initiating tramadol therapy in patients who are on a TCA, SNRI, or SSRI. There are several other medications administered in the inpatient setting that could also result in serotonin syndrome when co-administered with TCA including meperidine, chlorpheniramine, and linezolid.

Serotonin-Norepinephrine Reuptake Inhibitors

SNRIs work by inhibiting reuptake of serotonin and norepinephrine into the synaptic cleft, increasing the amount of available neurotransmitter at the nerve terminal. The mechanism by which SNRIs affect pain is thought to be through modulation of neurotransmission in descending inhibitory pain pathways [3]. SNRIs have been shown to have adverse effects on neurologic, cardiovascular, and gastrointestinal systems. Some of the more common adverse effects include insomnia, headache, hypertension, conduction abnormalities, nausea, dry mouth, dizziness, and constipation. Concurrent use of SNRIs and monoamine oxidase inhibitors (MAOIs) puts patients at risk for serotonin syndrome [3]. There is some evidence that suggests SNRIs may have a role in treating pain in the peri-operative period, but evidence is lacking.

Duloxetine

Duloxetine is approved in the United States for treatment of pain in diabetic peripheral neuropathy, fibromyalgia, and chronic musculoskeletal pain. In addition to impacting the central nervous system, duloxetine also modulates pain via the peripheral nervous system by blocking voltage-gated sodium channels [3]. Duloxetine should not be used in patients with clinically significant liver disease, renal failure, or uncontrolled narrow angle glaucoma, and should be avoided in patients with recent alcohol use disorder [3, 4].

Milnacipran

Milnacipran is approved in the United States for the treatment of chronic pain in fibromyalgia (Shelton 2018). Milnacipran likely affects pain via the central nervous system similar to duloxetine. Studies suggest that doses of 100 mg or 200 mg daily (in divided doses twice a day) have been shown to be effective in treating pain in some patients with fibromyalgia, while a majority of patients gain no clinically relevant benefit [3, 4]. Milnacipran has not been shown to be beneficial in treating neuropathic pain.

Venlafaxine/Desvenlafaxine

Venlafaxine and desvenlafaxine (the primary metabolite of venlafaxine) are not approved in the United States for the treatment of pain syndromes [3]. While historically included in pain regimens, more recent studies present conflicting evidence as to whether venlafaxine or desvenlafaxine have any efficacy in treating fibromyalgia or neuropathic pain [4]. For both of these drugs, hypertension is more common at higher doses, and the dosages should be reduced in patients with renal or hepatic impairment.

Continuation as Inpatient

For patients who take TCAs or SNRIs chronically on an outpatient basis, care should be taken to ensure that these medications are continued while inpatient if possible. Patients who stop taking antidepressant class medications suddenly are at risk for antidepressant discontinuation syndrome (ADS). Symptoms of ADS have typical onset of 1–7 days after medication discontinuation, and symptoms include dizziness, paresthesias, agitation, insomnia, nausea, vomiting, headache, confusion, and mood changes [5]. Chronic pain consultants should review outpatient medication lists to ensure that these medications are continued while the patient is admitted as an inpatient. There is no evidence to support initiating these medications as an inpatient, and, in fact, doing so may be deleterious to accurate dosing and titration.

References

1. Sindrup SH, Otto M, Finnerup NB, Jensen TS. Antidepressants in the treatment of neuropathic pain. Basic Clin Pharmacol Toxicol. 2005;96(6):399–409.
2. Reid IC, Stewart CA. How antidepressants work: New perspectives on the pathophysiology of depressive disorder. Br J Psychiatry. 2001;178(4):299–303.
3. Shelton RC. Serotonin and norepinephrine reuptake inhibitors. Handb Exp Pharmacol. 2018:1–36.

4. Welsch P, Üçeyler N, Klose P, Walitt B, Häuser W. Serotonin and noradrenaline reuptake inhibitors (SNRIs) for fibromyalgia. Cochrane Database Syst Rev. 2018;2(2):CD010292.
5. Bainum TB, Fike DS, Mechelay D, Haase KK. Effect of abrupt discontinuation of antidepressants in critically ill hospitalized adults. pharmacotherapy. J Hum Pharmacol Drug Therap. 2017;37(10):1231–40.

Steroids

36

Puneet Mishra, Lauren Poe, and Katherine Williams

Endogenous Steroids

Corticosteroids can be classified into three categories: glucocorticoids, mineralocorticoids, and androgens. Classically, the Hypothalamic-Pituitary-Adrenal (HPA) Axis is described as the primary production site of corticosteroids. The hypothalamus directs release of adrenocorticotropic hormone (ACTH) from the anterior pituitary, and ACTH stimulates adrenal cortex production of corticosteroids. The HPA axis is controlled via negative feedback mechanisms influenced by products of the adrenal cortex.

Aldosterone, the major mineralocorticoid, functions in regulating blood pressure, electrolytes and water. Androgens are responsible for masculinization or feminization of an individual and neurologic development. Most relevant to pain modulation, glucocorticoids, or cortisol, are released in response to stress. Their mechanisms are designed for blood pressure maintenance, immunomodulation, metabolism, regulating sleep/wake cycles, and decreased bone formation. Although classified by primary function, corticosteroids and their intermediate reactants may have some degree of cross reactivity within the other functional pathways.

Role of Steroids in Pain

Pain is mediated at the cellular level by a variety of signals in the central and peripheral nervous systems including glutamate, substance P, prostaglandins, bradykinin, serotonin, GABA, eicosanoids, endorphins, calcitonin gene related peptide, and

P. Mishra · L. Poe (✉)
Department of Anesthesiology, Vanderbilt University Medical Center, Nashville, TN, USA
e-mail: puneet.mishra@vumc.org; lauren.m.poe@vumc.org

K. Williams
Commonwealth Pain and Spine, Evansville, IN, USA
e-mail: kwilliams@mypainsolution.com

© Springer Nature Switzerland AG 2022
D. A. Edwards et al. (eds.), *Hospitalized Chronic Pain Patient*,
https://doi.org/10.1007/978-3-031-08376-1_36

Table 36.1 Diseases and injuries that benefit from steroids as adjunctive pain medicine

Low back pain: discogenic pain, radiculopathy
Inflammatory bowel disease: Crohn's disease, Ulcerative colitis
Autoimmune disease: Systemic lupus erythematosus, rheumatoid arthritis, myositis, Raynaud's, psoriasis
Trauma
Gout
Diabetes, Charcot-Marie-Tooth, spinal stenosis, neuropathic pain
Cancer: bone pain, malaise, fatigue, nausea, decreased appetite, liver capsular pain
Intracranial hypertension: headache
Asthma/COPD: pleuritic pain

free radicals [1]. These signals are produced through a variety of mechanisms including tissue injury, malignancy, paraneoplastic syndromes, and environmental stimuli. By utilizing steroid functions in cell-signaling and downstream processes, steroids can be used to treat a multitude of painful ailments (Table 36.1).

Inflammatory Pain

Typically, the result of cellular injury, inflammation stimulates nociceptive pathways leading to pain perception. Tissue injury results in subsequent release of inflammatory mediators as a means of initiating the immune response and the healing process. The principal role of glucocorticoids in modulating the pain process is through anti-inflammatory mechanisms. Pro-inflammatory cytokines cause vasodilation, leukocyte migration and increased vascular permeability. Steroids modify this process via binding to the Glucocorticoid Response Element in DNA which either represses or activates gene transcription by controlling transcription regulators [2].

Lymphocytes, neutrophils and mast cells migrate to the damaged area and produce signals for chemotaxis of more cells and vasodilation of blood vessels for increased release of substances to the area. Phospholipase A2, the major enzyme in the arachidonic acid pathway, results in the production of prostaglandins and leukotrienes, which contribute to edema by increasing vascular permeability in addition to functioning as painful signals [1]. Glucocorticoids stimulate the synthesis of lipocortin which inhibits phospholipase A2 and therefore the production of prostaglandin and leukotrienes [2]. Histamine causes vasodilation of blood vessels also contributing to edema and swelling; steroids block histamine release from mast cells. These cumulative effects result in significant reduction in edema. This makes steroids particularly useful in patients with Liver capsular pain, spinal cord compression, radiculopathy, neuropathy and headache from increased intracranial pressure [3].

Steroids hinder leukocyte adhesion and IL-2 production thus decreasing T cell proliferation and chemotaxis. These immunosuppressive effects decrease the degree of cytokine signaling and immune cell accumulation which contribute to inflammation and painful transmission (Table 36.2) [1]. These effects are the basis for steroid use in allergies, inflammatory and autoimmune diseases such as rheumatoid arthritis, gout, lupus, COPD, asthma, ulcerative colitis, and Crohn's disease.

Table 36.2 Steroids functions and effects

Anti-inflammatory	Hemodynamic	Metabolism
Inhibition of: • IL-2 (T cell proliferation) • Histamine release from mast cells • Eosinophils and basophils • Leukocyte adhesion • Prostaglandin/ leukotriene synthesis	• Upregulation of alpha 1 receptors • Increased sensitivity to catecholamines • Increased sodium reabsorption • Restoration of blood volume	Gluconeogenesis: • Enhanced protein catabolism • Increased lipolysis • Decreased insulin sensitivity • Decreased glucose utilization Bone resorption: • Inhibition of calcium uptake in GI tract

Neuropathic Pain

Neuropathic pain is characterized by burning, tingling, stabbing pain caused by inappropriate firing of a damaged nerve. Nerve damage may occur due to diabetes, trauma, malignancy, surgery, radiation or chemotherapeutic agents. Steroids have been shown to suppress ectopic discharges from a nerve and block signaling to the pro-inflammatory cytokine receptors of the endoneurium [1]. Steroids can also modulate nociceptive transmissions via effects on signaling in the central nervous system [1]. Steroids are lipophilic molecules and therefore pass through cell membranes, nerve sheaths and the blood-brain barrier. This is the basis for perineural injection as well as parenteral administration of steroids.

Steroids in Cancer and Associated Conditions

Cancer patients often experience anorexia, nausea, fatigue, and weight loss secondary to their disease process or medical therapies. Bone and visceral pain are also common in patients with malignancy. Steroids are recommended as adjunctive treatment for these symptoms as well as a variety of nonspecific cancer related symptoms and have been shown to improve overall quality of life [4, 5].

Administration

The etiology and acuity of the pain should dictate the manner of usage. Steroids may be administered by many routes: oral, parenteral, intra-articular, epidural, perineural, topical, or by inhalation. Oral agents available include dexamethasone, fludrocortisone and prednisone. For acute and highly painful syndromes, high oral dosing for 1–3 weeks can be appropriate. For cancer patients with visceral pain who need long-term therapy, a lower dosage may be used with fewer side effects. For those patients with pain along a nerve distribution, perineural injection may be the best treatment option.

Table 36.3 Side effects of steroids

Common	Long-term usage	Serious or Life-threatening
Hyperglycemia	Infection	Gastrointestinal bleeding
Insomnia	Cushing syndrome	Thromboembolism
Weight gain/increased appetite	Adrenal suppression	Aseptic necrosis of bone
Mood disturbance/Psychosis	Proximal myopathy	Bone fractures
Acne	Neuropathy	Pancreatitis
Elevated blood pressure	Osteoporosis	

Side Effects

There are a variety of side effects of corticosteroids (Table 36.3) that may preclude them from being used as a long-term therapy for pain [3–5]. Adverse effects can depend on the length of use and dosage; therefore, it is suggested to use steroids for the shortest amount of time possible to achieve maximal benefit. HPA axis suppression is a concern with acute withdrawal of steroids. Therefore, tapering may be required if steroids need to be discontinued or stress dose steroids may be indicated in the acute care setting. Tapering strategy and stress dosing plans are dose-dependent and driven by duration of use.

References

1. Benzon H. Essentials of pain medicine. 4th ed. Philadelphia, PA: Elsevier; 2018.
2. Rijsdijk M, vanWijck AJ, Kalkman CJ, Yaksh TL. The effects of glucocorticoids on neuropathic pain: a review with emphasis on intrathecal methylprednisolone acetate delivery. Anesth Analg. 2014;118:1097–112.
3. Vyvey M. Steroids as pain relief adjuvants. Can Fam Physician. 2010;56(12):1295–7.
4. Leppert W, Buss T. The role of corticosteroids in the treatment of pain in cancer patients. Curr Pain Headache Rep. 2012;16(4):307–13.
5. Lussier D, Huskey AG, Portenoy RK. Adjuvant analgesics in cancer pain management. Oncologist. 2004;9(5):571–91.

Cannabinoids

37

Christopher M. Sobey, Hai Nguyen, and Greg Carpenter

Background

There are multiple derivatives from the cannabis plant that have uses in medical treatment. These are called cannabinoids, which are lipid compounds that target G-coupled protein receptors throughout the body. Three major categories of cannabinoids exist—phytocannabinoids (derived from plants), endocannabinoids, and synthetic compounds [1]. The two primary receptors for cannabinoids are CB1 and CB2. CB1 is found mostly within the central nervous system and it responsible primarily for the psychotropic and euphoric effects of cannabinoids. The receptor acts at the pre-synaptic junction to inhibit the release of excitatory neurotransmitters including NE, acetylcholine, glutamate and dopamine. CB2 is found mostly in the periphery as well as on immune cells and is thought to play a role in the regulation of inflammatory states [2].

The most noted compound derived from cannabis is THC (tetrahydrocannabinol), which is the most intoxicating substance from the plant and is primarily responsible for the psychotropic effects of cannabis [1]. Ingestion of THC causes the greatest down-regulation of the body's own endogenous cannabinoid receptors. Positively, it is thought to have antioxidant properties that are neuroprotective from glutamate excitation.

An agent that has gained much popularity in our culture both medically and societally is CBD or cannabidiol, It is considered less intoxicating than THC,

C. M. Sobey (✉)
Department of Anesthesiology, Vanderbilt University Medical Center, Nashville, TN, USA
e-mail: christopher.m.sobey@vumc.org

H. Nguyen
Minivasive Pain and Orthopedics, Spring, TX, USA

G. Carpenter
Department of Anesthesiology, VA Tennessee Valley Healthcare System, Nashville, TN, USA

© Springer Nature Switzerland AG 2022
D. A. Edwards et al. (eds.), *Hospitalized Chronic Pain Patient*,
https://doi.org/10.1007/978-3-031-08376-1_37

however, it has the potential to increase THC plasma concentrations and reduce plasma clearance. It is believed to have many properties to include anti-inflammatory, anti-epileptic and a potential maintenance medication for those with histories of drug abuse and overall counteract the negative effects of THC itself [1]. To note, it acts as an indirect antagonist at the cannabinoid receptors [2].

In Europe and Asia there has been an increase in the use of nabiximols, derived from the sativa cannabis strain they are a mixture of CBD and THC and is targeted for patients with multiple sclerosis (MS) with specific complaints of spasticity, overactive bladder, and neuropathic pain syndromes [3]. It is currently undergoing phase III trials in the USA for the treatment of cancer related pain. It has already been approved in Canada for the treatment of MS and neuropathic pain states.

Synthetically derived cannabinoids include the FDA approved dronabinol. It is a pure isomer of THC that is sold in capsule formulary (previously as a resin in oil suspension). It was initially intended to be used as an anti-emetic for patients with refractory nausea related to chemotherapy for cancer and as an appetite stimulant for severe anorexia, especially those suffering from HIV/AIDS [3, 4]. It was downgraded from a schedule I drug to a schedule II in 1986 and then further downgraded to schedule III in 1999 according to the Controlled Substances Act. It has also been used in patients with MS and seizure disorders [3]. Its common side effects include abdominal pain, euphoria, sedation, worsening nausea and vomiting, change in cognition and cognitive abilities making it often times intolerable for many patients [5, 6].

Multiple studies have been performed on various types of chronic pain conditions using cannabis-derived products (Table 37.1). Much of this evidence is based on studies with many confounders or moderate-to-low quality analyses. The strongest evidence for use is on cancer pain, but there is promising evidence for non-malignant chronic pain and neuropathic pain [1, 2, 10]. No consensus has been determined on dosing or standardized regimen; however, higher doses are associated with greater side effects (most notably sedation). Given dearth of high-quality studies, would recommend as a last line of a multimodal approach or continuing if already on stable outpatient regimen.

Public and Mental Health Concerns

Cannabinoids is quickly emerging into its own drug class (Table 37.2). With the push towards uniform legality, there will undoubtedly be more research produced in the field. Important aspects that should be scrutinized include cannabinoid effects on mental health (i.e. depression, anxiety, suicidal ideation and psychosis), addiction, driving while under the influence of cannabinoids and cannabis as a strategy to improve outcomes under medical supervision versus recreational use.

The primary issue that providers currently face is the lack of quality scientific studies. Other concerns include unregulated cannabinoid products on the market, impurities of products leading to positive drug screens and their ramifications,

Table 37.1 Types of pain and cannabinoid use [3, 5, 7–9]

	Cancer pain is the most researched clinical use for cannabinoids with evidence for some significant analgesic effects		
Cancer pain	Compound	Description	Use
	Tetrahydrocannabinol (THC)	One of the three phytocannabinoids found in the cannabis plant, along with cannabidiol (CBD) and cannabinol (CBN). Main source of psychotropic effects	10–20 mg PO used for pain adjuncts. Equivalent to 60–120 mg of codeine. Increased dosage results in limiting side effects of sedation and confusion
	Nabiximols	Oromucosal spray of THC and CBD. Common dosage in each spray equates to 2.7 mg of THC and 2.5 mg CBD (variable formulations)	Self-titrated use by patients with poor pain control with opiates alone can lead up to a 30% improvement in pain scores. Does not reduce median dose of opiates, nausea or sleep scores
Neuropathic pain	Compound	Description	Use
	Ajulemic acid	Synthetic derivative of a THC metabolite. Shows promise with analgesic and anti-inflammatory profile without psychotropic effects	Doses of 40–80 mg BID have shown significant reduction in pain scores. Common side effects include dry mouth, tiredness, and dizziness
	Nabiximols	Superior to placebo in pain reduction and sleep disturbance reduction measures	Self-titrated use of oromucosal spray. Average number of sprays per patient approximately 9.6/day
	THC	Promising evidence in reduction of HIV-induced and posttraumatic neuropathic pain. Overall reduction of pain and increase in sleep quality	Study using self-titrated use of 3.56% THC cigarettes. Side effects included difficulty concentrating, sedation, fatigue, increased number of sleep hours, thirst
Acute pain	Compound	Description	Use
	Cannador	Oral capsule of cannabis plant extract with THC to CBD ratio of 2:1. Used in postsurgical patients with continued pain after stopping PCA post-surgery	Usual dosages 5mg to 15mg q6h PRN leads to decreased need for rescue analgesic Significant side effects include sedation and vasovagal events

(continued)

Table 37.1 (continued)

	Cancer pain is the most researched clinical use for cannabinoids with evidence for some significant analgesic effects		
Cancer pain	Compound	Description	Use
Chronic pain	Compound	Description	Use
	Dronabinol	Pure isomer of THC. Shows promise in reducing pain and increasing satisfaction of chronic pain patients of all types of chronic pain	5 mg daily to 20 mg TID dosing. Side effects include anxiety, sedation, drowsiness, dry mouth, confusion
	Nabiximols	Oromucosal spray of THC and CBD	Self-titrated oral spray showed improvement in pain and quality of sleep

Table 37.2 Common cannabinoids and dosing

Common cannabinoids and dosing	
Drug	Usual dosing
THC	Inhaled: Self titrated 3.56% cigarettes PRN
	PO: 10–20 mg Q4-8H PRN pain
Dronabinol	PO: 5 mg daily up to 20 mg TID as tolerated
Cannador	PO 5–15 mg q6H PRN
Nabiximol	PO: Self titrate oromucosal spray. Usual composition—2.7 mg of THC and 2.5 mg CBD per spray
Ajulemic acid	20–40 mg BID

public misinformation, interference with metabolism of other medications and unknown long-term effects of chronic use. As more data is collected and analyzed, there will be a better understanding of the safety and efficacy of this drug class.

References

1. Mucke M, Phillips T, Radbruch L, et al. Cannabis-based medicines for chronic neuropathic pain in adults. Cochrane Database Syst Rev. 2018;3:CD012182.
2. Johnson JR, Burnell-Nugent M, Lossignol D, et al. Multicenter, double-blind, randomized, placebo-controlled, parallel-group study of the efficacy, safety, and tolerability of THC: CBD extract and THC extract in patients with intractable cancer-related pain. J Pain Symptom Manag. 2010;39(2):167–79.
3. Whiting PF, Wolff RF, Deshpande S, et al. Cannabinoids for medical use: a systematic review and meta-analysis. JAMA. 2015;313(24):2456–73.
4. Abrams DI, Jay CA, Shade SB, et al. Cannabis in painful HIV-associated sensory neuropathy: a randomized placebo-controlled trial. Neurology. 2007;68(7):515–21.
5. Narang S, Gibson D, Wasan AD, et al. Efficacy of dronabinol as an adjuvant treatment for chronic pain patients on opioid therapy. J Pain. 2008;9(3):254–64.
6. Ware MA, Wang T, Shapiro S, et al. Smoked cannabis for chronic neuropathic pain: a randomized controlled trial. CMAJ. 2010;182(14):694–701.

7. Holdcroft A, Maze M, Dore C, Tebbs S, Thompson S. A multicenter dose-escalation study of the analgesic and adverse effects of an oral cannabis extract (Cannador) for postoperative pain management. Anesthesiology. 2006;104(5):1040–6.
8. Karst M, Salim K, Burstein S, et al. Analgesic effect of the synthetic cannabinoid CT-3 on chronic neuropathic pain. JAMA. 2003;290(13):1757–62.
9. Smith F, Cicheqicz D, Martin ZL, Welch SP. The enhancement of morphine antinociception in mice by delta9-tetrahydrocannabinol. Pharmacol Biochem Behav. 1998;60(2):559–66.
10. Meng H, Johnston B, Englesakis M, Moulin DE, Bhatia A. Selective cannabinoids for chronic neuropathic pain: a systematic review and meta-analysis. Anesth Analg. 2017;125(5):1638–52.

Part V

Interventional Treatments

Peripheral Regional Anesthesia Blocks

38

Vikram Bansal

Introduction

There are basic rules for a safe regional anesthesia practice. An in-depth knowledge of anatomy, procedural skills, sterile technique are some key elements to be. respected. There are many resources that are available online to aid our regional skills, including the New York School of Regional Anesthesia (www.nysora.com) and the Military Advanced Regional Anesthesia and Analgesia handbook (www. dvcipm.org).

Having the proper equipment and ancillary staff is vital to a successful regional service. With the advent of ultrasonography, regional anesthesia has become safer with a faster onset, higher success rates and fewer needle passes as compared to nerve stimulation [1]. Ultrasonography guided regional anesthesia has become the standard of care (Tables 38.1, 38.2, and 38.3). Even with advances in technique and technology, chronic pain patients remain a difficult population to manage.

Regional anesthesia is an excellent option for chronic pain patients due to its mechanism of action and its ability to alleviate pain independent of any pain medication regimen or chronic pain states. However, there are limits to the duration of regional anesthesia and there are rare reports of local anesthetic resistance in chronic

Table 38.1 Upper extremity and regional techniques

Location of procedure/pain	Brachial plexus approach
Shoulder/upper humerus/distal clavicle	Interscalene
Mid-lower humerus/arm/elbow/forearm/hand	Supraclavicular
Elbow/forearm/hand	Infraclavicular
Forearm/hand	Axillary

V. Bansal (✉)

Department of Anesthesiology, Vanderbilt University Medical Center, Nashville, TN, USA
e-mail: Vikram.bansal@vumc.org

© Springer Nature Switzerland AG 2022
D. A. Edwards et al. (eds.), *Hospitalized Chronic Pain Patient*,
https://doi.org/10.1007/978-3-031-08376-1_38

Table 38.2 Lower extremity and regional techniques

Location of procedure/pain	Regional approach
Hip	Lumbar plexus nerve block
Anterior thigh/knee	Femoral nerve block
Medial aspect of lower leg/foot	Saphenous nerve block
Posterior thigh/posterior knee/anterior lower leg/posterior lower leg/ankle/foot	Sciatic nerve block (transgluteal, subgluteal, anterior approach)
Anterior and posterior lower leg/ankle/foot	Popliteal approach to sciatic nerve block
Foot/metatarsals	Ankle block

Table 38.3 Truncal blocks

Location of procedure/pain	Regional approach
Chest	Thoracic epidural, paravertebral, intercostal nerve blocks, pectoral nerve blocks, erector spinae blocks
Abdomen	Low thoracic epidural, low paravertebral, quadratus lumborum block
	Transversus abdominus plane and/or rectus sheath block
Hip/knee	Lumbar epidural

Table 38.4 Common anticoagulants and regional anesthesia technique

	Single shot peripheral nerve blockade	Catheter placement peripheral nerve	Neuraxial
Heparin prophylaxis	Proceed	Wait 4 h after last dose	Wait 4 h after last dose
Heparin therapeutic (infusion)	No guidelines, use your clinical judgment	Avoid	Avoid
Lovenox prophylaxis	No guidelines-may proceed if superficial block	Wait 12 h after last dose	Wait 12 h after last dose
Lovenox therapeutic	No guidelines-may proceed if superficial block	Wait 24 h after last dose	Wait 24 h after last dose
Warfarin	No guidelines-may proceed if superficial block	INR <1.5	INR <1.5

pain patients [2]. Single bolus injections with adjunctive components or perineural catheters may be placed to prolong duration of analgesia. A transition from a continuous catheter to oral medications to maintain analgesia following discontinuation of infusion is recommended for patients with heightened sensitivity due to underlying chronic pain. It is important to continue a patient's chronic pain regimen, in order to avoid withdrawal and decompensation when the blocks fade. Regional analgesia provides many benefits for the chronic pain patient including improved patient satisfaction, increased safety in patients with multiple comorbidities and decreased opioid use in both acute and chronic settings [3]. Moreover, complicating issues of hyperalgesia and increasing tolerance to opioids can be mitigated with effective regional anesthesia [4].

Importantly, appropriate patient selection is key to the successful treatment of any patient with regional anesthesia. Patients with an active infection or anticoagulation may be contraindicated to regional anesthesia (Table 38.4). The location of pain is also of key importance, as different peripheral nerve blocks provide different analgesic coverage. Chronic pain patients may require additional sedation during regional procedures in the setting of heightened anxiety and warrant an in-depth discussion of expectations and the possibility of failure and/or incomplete coverage [3, 4]. In addition, a comprehensive discussion of the risks and benefits is extremely important and may alleviate patient concerns. Regional anesthesia has the potential to reduce chronic pain associated with surgery and/or trauma, a major benefit to chronic pain patients who may be more prone to such conditions [5]. Patient follow up is required until regional analgesia has subsided, and paresthesia resolved to ensure no nerve injury occurred during placement. If paresthesia continues and a nerve injury is suspected, proper follow up with the patient's surgeon, a neurologist and further neurological testing may be warranted. It is important, as the anesthesiologist, to remain in contact with the patient as well to provide guidance, reassurance, and expertise when warranted.

Complications/Precautions

Major risks involved in regional analgesia for a chronic pain patient are similar to those of other patient populations. Risks include bleeding, infection, damage to local structures and nerve injury. Transient paresthesia may occur in relation to blunt trauma, stretch, compression, drug neurotoxicity or nerve ischemia, of which, 99% resolve within a year. However, it is believed that patients with pre-existing neuropathy are at greatest risk for paresthesia, which may include a subset of chronic pain patients [6]. Other complications include seizure, cardiovascular collapse, dysrhythmias and local anesthetic systemic toxicity. These are serious but rare complications often associated with an intravascular injection of local anesthetic or rapid systemic absorption.

- Please use your clinical judgment and weigh the potential risks and benefits of each block (Table 38.5).
- Potential risks are higher with neuraxial procedures, such as an epidural hematoma which can result in catastrophic consequences such as paralysis.
- Superficial peripheral nerve blockade may be acceptable even with anticoagulation due to the ability to compress any bleeding.

Table 38.5 Benefits of utilizing regional anesthesia [4]

In chronic pain patient	Opioid Sparing
	Better pain control with increased patient satisfaction
	Chronic post-operative pain prevention
In all patients	All three above
	Decreased surgical stress in patients with other co-morbidities
	Decreased stress response in cancer patients
	Decreased hospital length of stay
	Improved post-operative mobility
	Potentially lower risk of cognitive dysfunction in children or elderly patients

- Deeper blocks such as sciatic, lumbar plexus or complicated regional techniques such as a paravertebral block should be treated more conservatively like neuraxial procedures.
- There are many new anticoagulants prescribed to patients and very few studies exist that look at complication rates with peripheral nerve blockade.
- Please consult the American Society of Regional Anesthesia and Pain Medicine (ASRA) practice advisory for further information about these and other anticoagulants (www.asra.com/advisory-guidelines).

References

1. Abrahams MS, Aziz MF, Fu RF, Horn JL. Ultrasound guidance compared with electrical neurostimulation for peripheral nerve block: a systematic review and meta-analysis of randomized controlled trials. Br J Anaesth. 2009;102:408–17.
2. Chou R, et al. Guidelines on the management of postoperative pain. Management of postoperative pain: a clinical practice guideline from the American Pain Society, the American Society of Regional Anesthesia and Pain Medicine, and the American Society of Anesthesiologists' Committee on Regional Anesthesia, Executive Committee, and Administrative Council. J Pain. 2016;17:131–57.
3. Souzdalnitski D, et al. Regional anesthesia and co-existing chronic pain. Curr Opin Anaesthesiol. 2010;23:662–70.
4. Rivat C, et al. Mechanisms of regional anaesthesia protection against hyperalgesia and pain chronicization. Curr Opin Anaesthesiol. 2013;26:621–5.
5. Andreae MH, et al. Local anaesthetics and regional anaesthesia for preventing chronic pain after surgery. Cochrane Libr. 2012;10:CD007105.
6. Sorenson EJ. Neurological injuries associated with regional anesthesia. Reg Anesth Pain Med. 2008;33:442–8.

Neuraxial Blocks

39

Eugene Leytin and Brian F. S. Allen

Anatomy

The human vertebral column is comprised of 7 cervical, 12 thoracic, 5 lumbar, 5 fused sacral, and 4 fused coccygeal vertebrae. Ligaments connect the vertebrae in a way that provide support but allow vertebrae to bend, twist, and move in relation to each other. Inside the vertebral canal sits the thecal sac, spinal cord, roots, and cerebrospinal fluid (CSF). Outside of the thecal sac is the epidural space, containing fat and blood vessels. Spinal roots emerge at each vertebral level and travel peripherally relaying sensory information and motor impulses. Neuraxial procedures take advantage of this anatomy to provide segmental analgesia or anesthesia. Neuraxial procedures involve delivery of local anesthetic (LA) or other medications into the epidural or intrathecal spaces.

Midline epidurals traverse the following structures in order: skin, subcutaneous fat, supraspinous ligament, interspinous ligament, ligamentum flavum, and epidural space. The spinal cord normally ends at L1–L2 in adults (L2–L3 in children).

Technique

Prior to considering a neuraxial procedure for a particular patient, be aware of relative and absolute contraindications (Table 39.1).

Options for placement include lumbar, thoracic, caudal, or cervical epidural, lumbar spinal, or combined spinal epidural, The area affected by a neuraxial block depends on (1) vertebral level of placement, (2) intrathecal vs. epidural placement,

E. Leytin
Bend Anesthesiology Group, Bend, OR, USA

B. F. S. Allen (✉)
Department of Anesthesiology, Vanderbilt University Medical Center, Nashville, TN, USA
e-mail: Brian.allen@vumc.org

© Springer Nature Switzerland AG 2022
D. A. Edwards et al. (eds.), *Hospitalized Chronic Pain Patient*,
https://doi.org/10.1007/978-3-031-08376-1_39

Table 39.1
Contraindications to
neuraxial anesthesia

Contraindications
• Patient refusal
• Coagulopathy
• Anticoagulants and antiplatelet agents
• Elevated intracranial pressures
• Infection at the site of needle puncture
Relative contraindications
• Severe aortic stenosis
• LV outflow obstruction
• Severe mitral stenosis
• Sepsis/bacteremia
• Demyelinating disease

Table 39.2 Surface and
palpation landmarks For
neuraxial blockade [1]

C7 spinous process (SP)
• The vertebra prominens
• Distinguish from T1 SP by head rotation
• C7 SP should move with head rotation
• Most accurate landmark for identifying vertebral level
Tip of the Scapula
• Corresponds to the level of T7 SP
• Less accurate than using C7 SP
Intercristal Line
• Line connecting iliac crests
• Radiographically corresponds to L4–L5
• Line by palpation corresponds to L3–L4
Sacral Hiatus
• Palpated at the S4 level between the sacral cornua

(3) medications administered (agent(s), volume, concentration, baricity), and (4) patient factors (positioning and anatomic variation).

Monitors during placement should include pulse oximetry, ECG (preferred but not required), and blood pressure. Resuscitative medications and equipment should be readily available. The patient should be placed with the spine in flexion in the sitting, lateral decubitus, or prone position. Palpable landmarks can guide identification of the desired vertebral level (Table 39.2).

For neuraxial blockade, two needle approaches are available: midline or paramedian. The midline approach sagittal plane parallel to the spinous process. In contrast, the paramedian approach starts ~1 cm lateral to midline and approaches the epidural space obliquely, bypassing ligaments and only encountering Ligamentum flavum. This approach is useful in thoracic epidurals where SPs overlie one another at a steep angle.

A "loss of resistance" technique using a low-friction glass or plastic syringe is employed for epidural placement. When the Tuohy needle is engaged in ligament, the stylet is withdrawn and the syringe attached. When needle tip is in ligament, it is difficult to inject the contents of the syringe. Once the tip of the Tuohy passes the ligamentum flavum, entering the epidural space, there is a loss of resistance to injection. An indwelling catheter is threaded, the Tuohy withdrawn, and the catheter secured at the skin. Then a test dose of 45 mg lidocaine with 15 mcg epinephrine is given through the catheter to rule out intravascular or intrathecal (IT) injection. A rise in heart rate of approximately 20 beats/min, 20 seconds after injection, lasting for 20 seconds (rule of 20's) caused by epinephrine suggests intravascular injection. If intrathecal, leg weakness from the LA would occur rapidly.

Pharmacology

Neuraxial procedures often utilize local anesthetics (LA), with or without adjuncts such as opioids or alpha-adrenergic agents. LA selection is based on desired duration of action (Table 39.3).

Baricity of the LA (density of LA vs. the density of CSF) is an important consideration when selecting a spinal medication. Hyperbaric solutions placed IT are denser than CSF and will "sink" with gravity. LAs prepared with 5-8% dextrose will be hyperbaric. Hypobaric solutions, created by mixing LA in sterile water, will "rise" against gravity. An isobaric IT solution (made with saline) will stay roughly where deposited, with spread determined by dose. Adjuncts to LA can be used in the epidural or IT spaces, with the most common being opioids (morphine, fentanyl, hydromorphone, sufentanil, etc.) and alpha-adrenergic agents (epinephrine and clonidine). Neuraxial opioids can be potent analgesics via an opioid-receptor effect at the dorsal horn of the spinal cord [4]. This effect is potent even in patients tolerant to enteral or parenteral opioids, which have effects primarily on the brainstem. Thus, patients tolerant to enteral or parenteral opioids may benefit greatly from neuraxial opioids.

Physiological Response

Spinal and epidural LAs block not only sensory, but motor, sympathetic, and parasympathetic nerves. Decreases in sympathetic tone result in arterial and venous dilation and potential hypotension from decreased systemic vascular resistance and decreased preload to the right heart. Crystalloid co-administration (fluid bolus)

Table 39.3 Local anesthetics [2, 3]

Type	Spinal dose (mg)	Spinal resolution (SR) (min)	SR with 1:200k Epi (min)	Epidural dose (mg)	Epidural resolution (min)	Medication concentration (%)
Chloroprocaine	30–100	45–60	Do not use[a]	30–900	30–90	2–3
Lidocaine[b]	30–80	60–100	120–180	30–400	45–120	0.5–2
Mepivacaine[b]	40–60	90–140	140–200	30–400	60–180	1–2
Ropivacaine	5–20	140–180	150–200	10–200	240–420	0.2–1
Bupivacaine	5–15	160–220	180–240	6.25–175	300–460	0.25–0.5
Tetracaine	5–20	160–220	180–240		300–460	0.5–1

[a] The addition of epinephrine to spinal chloroprocaine may produce flu-like symptoms in patients
[b] Lidocaine and Mepivacaine are both historically associated with TNS (transient neurological symptoms)

during neuraxial anesthesia decreases hypotension, though utilization of vasopressors is also useful [5]. Phenylephrine, an alpha-1 agonist, and the sympathomimetic ephedrine are two commonly used vasoactive medications to manage hypotension during neuraxial anesthesia.

Side Effects and Complications

A high, or total, spinal is due to an excessively high level of neuraxial anesthetic resulting in phrenic nerve (C3–C5) blockade, apnea, potential cerebral hypoperfusion and loss of consciousness. Management is supportive, usually necessitating securing an airway and utilizing vasoactive medications for hemodynamic control.

Severe bradycardia may rarely occur, potentially causing asystole and cardiac arrest. Blockade of cardiac accelerator fibers at T1–T4 during higher levels of anesthesia is one proposed etiology of this effect.

Dural puncture may result in a postdural puncture headache (PDPH), either from unintentional dural puncture from a 17 or 18 gauge Tuohy needle, or less commonly intentional puncture during a spinal anesthetic. PDPH may cause nausea, diplopia, and/or other neurologic findings. It is likely caused by persistent CSF leak, leading to intracranial hypotension with traction on the meninges and nerves. The headache is postural: alleviated by lying flat, worsened by sitting or standing. Conservative treatment includes hydration, caffeine, and analgesics while epidural blood patch is the definitive therapy [6].

Epidural hematoma is a feared complication of neuraxial anesthesia. It occurs when epidural bleeding causes compression of the spinal cord or roots, causing ischemia associated with motor weakness, bladder sphincter dysfunction, lower extremity sensory loss, or back pain. Epidural hematoma requires urgent recognition and surgical evacuation to prevent irreversible neurologic injury. Epidural abscess or infection, another emergency, can present with similar symptoms as well as fever and more prominent back pain. Emergent spine MRI is indicated when abscess or hematoma are suspected [7]. Careful attention to a patient's anticoagulant and antiplatelet medications as well as coagulation status can minimize risk of hematoma. The American Society of Regional Anesthesia and Pain Medicine guidelines and decision support tools should guide appropriate management [8].

Transient neurological symptoms, associated with lidocaine or rarely mepivacaine spinal anesthesia, present as severe low back or radicular pain without sensory or motor deficits and is self-limited. Urinary retention, pruritis, lower extremity weakness, and other various side effects are possible with epidural local anesthetics or opioids.

Conclusion

A number of neuraxial techniques are available to aid pain control in the hospitalized patient. Local anesthetics and opioids administered epidurally or intrathecally are potent analgesics that can provide superior pain control, even to opioid tolerant individuals. Careful use of these techniques, while remaining cognizant of the risks, is an excellent option in the chronic pain patient.

References

1. Shin S, Yoon DM, Yoon KB. Identification of the correct cervical level by palpation of spinous processes. Anesth Analg. 2011;112(5):1232–5.
2. Barash PG. Clinical anesthesia. 7th ed. Philadelphia: Wolters Kluwer Health; 2013.
3. Panesar K. Epidural anesthesia during labor and delivery. US Pharm. 2014;29(3):11–4.
4. Bernards CM. Recent insights into the pharmacokinetics of spinal opioids and the relevance to opioid selection. Curr Opin Anaesthesiol. 2004;17(5):441–7.
5. Teoh WHL, Sia ATH. Colloid preload versus coload for spinal anesthesia for cesarean delivery: the effects on maternal cardiac output. Anesth Analg. 2009;108(5):1592–8.
6. Gaiser RR. Postdural puncture headache. Anesthesiol Clin. 2017;35(1):157–67.
7. Bateman BT, Mhyre JM, Ehrenfeld J, et al. The risk and outcomes of epidural hematomas after perioperative and obstetric epidural catheterization. Anesth Analg. 2013;116(6):1380–5.
8. Horlocker TT, Vandermeuelen E, Kopp SL, et al. Regional anesthesia in the patient receiving antithrombotic or thrombolytic therapy. Reg Anesth Pain Med. 2018;43(3):263–309.

Vertebroplasty and Kyphoplasty

Brandon Gish and Daniel Lonergan

Background

Patients with VCF and persistent pain, despite conservative management, may be candidates for percutaneous vertebroplasty (PVP) or balloon kyphoplasty (BKP). Conservative management generally includes back bracing, physical therapy, multimodal oral analgesics (NSAIDs, acetaminophen, muscle relaxers), and therapy guided to the underlying cause such as treatment of osteoporosis. The time frame for pursuing conservative therapy is generally accepted to be approximately 6 weeks [1].

PVP is the percutaneous injection of polymethylmethacrylate (PMMA) into a fractured vertebral body. BKP is the inflation of a balloon into a VCF to restore height loss followed by injection of PMMA into the fracture and void created by the balloon. These are generally performed under light sedation and can be performed in a clinic, ASC, or hospital setting. Cement injection is thought to have analgesic benefit by stabilizing mobile fractures, reducing mechanical stress associated with activity and weight, and painful nerve endings are thought to be destroyed during cement polymerization by exothermic and cytotoxic reactions [2].

Literature Review

The Canadian Multicentre Osteoporosis Study reported that 21.5% of women and 23.5% of men >50 years old have at least 1 vertebral compression deformity and a Norwegian based population study found 20.3% of males and 19.2% of females

B. Gish (✉)
Commonwealth Pain and Spine, Lexington, KY, USA

D. Lonergan
Cuyuna Regional Medical Center, Crosby, MN, USA

© Springer Nature Switzerland AG 2022
D. A. Edwards et al. (eds.), *Hospitalized Chronic Pain Patient*,
https://doi.org/10.1007/978-3-031-08376-1_40

have at least one vertebral compression fracture (VCF). Despite this high prevalence, nearly two thirds remain undiagnosed [1]. Common causes of VCF are osteoporosis, cancer, radionecrosis, and trauma.

Some evidence suggests that early vertebroplasty (prior to a 6-week time frame of conservative management) may be beneficial in reducing pain from >7/10 to <4/10 when compared to control patients; however, at the time of writing many insurance carriers require 6 weeks of conservative therapy prior to more invasive procedures.

Initial excitement in PVP and BKP was criticized by two SHAM studies in the NEJM [3, 4], which showed no significant benefit of PVP over SHAM procedure in VCF due to osteoporosis. Critics of these studies point to the small sample size, allowed crossover, chronicity of many of the fractures analyzed (average 9–18 weeks), and inconsistent use of MRI bone edema as inclusion criteria [5]. Despite these criticisms, it should be recognized that with time patients in the conservative arm did have improved pain, proposed to be timed with fracture healing.

Subsequent studies have compared conservative treatment with BKP with mean fracture duration of approximately 5–6 weeks. An industry sponsored study showed significant improvement in the BKP group at 1 month, with diminished differences at 12 months. There was not an increased rate of subsequent fracture in the BKP group compared to conservative management [6]. These results were repeated for vertebroplasty in a similar study of fractures less than 6 weeks old in patients with pain >5/10 VAS; however, pain relief was significantly improved even out to one year, with significant reduction in medication usage in the vertebroplasty arm [5].

Much recent research has focused on osteoporotic vertebral compression fractures, but similar positive results have been found for cancer related vertebral fractures. Pain, functionality, and quality of life are significantly improved with early kyphoplasty over conservative treatment up to 1 year, with no increased risk of subsequent vertebral fractures [7]. However, just as is the case for osteoporotic compression fractures, patients may have multiple pain generators in the spine aside from a compression fracture. It also may be likely that multiple vertebral compressions are present, in which case kyphoplasty to one body will likely be insufficient.

Importantly, retrospective data from large Medicare cohorts (2005–2009), showed improved mortality and morbidity in those that underwent vertebral augmentation procedures (BKP or PVP) than those treated conservatively, with a 19% lower adjusted risk of mortality for BKP over PVP [8].

Treatments and Care Plan [1]

Conservative management

- Thoracolumbar support bracing
- Physical therapy
- Medication management: acetaminophen, NSAIDs, opioids

Indications for proceeding with vertebroplasty or kyphoplasty:

- Level of pain >4/10
- Unable to ambulate or do physical activities
- Negative side effects from pain medications
- Pain location matches with MRI findings
- Edema on MRI (T2 weighted STIR sequence)
- Height loss, deformity (controversial)

Balloon kyphoplasty procedure:

- Transpedicular approach vs. extrapedicular approach vs. en face approach
- Obtain bone biopsy in the setting of cancer history
- Unilateral vs. bilateral technique

Osteoporosis treatment

- DEXA study
- Vitamin D
- Calcitonin for short duration
- Bisphosphonates

Multidisciplinary Approach and Considerations

Given the complexity of treating compression fractures it is vital to have a multidisciplinary approach to overall care. If the etiology is assumed to be osteoporosis this should confirmed with a DEXA scan and appropriate medical treatment outlined by either a primary care provider or subspecialist. Similarly, if the etiology is from cancer, close communication with the oncology team can help guide the use of chemotherapy and radiation options in management.

Case Result

Given the atraumatic nature of painful episode which did not include a fall, the most likely etiology is underlying osteoporosis. An MRI should confirm that this is an acute fracture (findings of marrow edema on STIR sequences).

The patient should begin conservative therapy including back bracing, physical therapy, and limited axial loading. Total bed rest should be avoided as this increases risk for the development of DVT and pulmonary complications. A DEXA scan can confirm the presence of osteoporosis and a referral should be made to her primary physician or sub-specialist for ongoing management.

Once an adequate duration of conservative therapy has been trialed (approximately 4–6 weeks) she may be evaluated as a candidate for vertebral augmentation.

With absence of improvement in pain, VAS >4/10, and impaired functionality, she may consider moving forward with vertebral augmentation. This is an elective procedure. The patient should be counseled that, if given enough time, the fracture will heal and pain may improve, however in the several months following a fracture, severe pain can be improved more quickly with the use of BKP or PVP. Pain may be improved with BKP and/or PVP for up to 12 months compared to more conservative therapy. In addition, epidemiological data suggests that adjusted risk of mortality may be greater by opting for conservative therapy rather than performing BKP.

Other interventions for low back pain may also be considered, such as epidural steroid injections or medial branch workup and radiofrequency ablation for axial facet loading pain.

Summary

- Vertebral compression fractures (VCFs) are a common consequence of patients with osteoporosis.
- Once an osteoporotic VCF has occurred, there is a fivefold risk for VCFs at other levels.
- Untreated VCFs can be associated with chronic pain, neurologic complications, and decreased mobility which can confer a higher risk of mortality.
- Treatment with vertebral augmentation in the subacute phase of a VCF can improve pain and quality of life in the months following the fracture.

References

1. Kendler A, et al. Vertebral fractures: clinical importance and management. Am J Med. 2016;129:2.
2. Wang A, et al. Comparison of percutaneous vertebroplasty and balloon kyphoplasty for the treatment of single level vertebral fractures: a meta-analysis of the literature. Pain Physician. 2015;18:209–11.
3. Buchbinder A, et al. A randomized trial of vertebroplasty for painful osteoporotic vertebral fractures. NEJM. 2009;361:9.
4. Kallmes A, et al. A randomized trial of vertebroplasty for osteoporotic vertebral fractures. NEJM. 2009;361:569–79.
5. Klazen A, et al. Vertebroplasty versus conservative treatment in acute osteoporotic vertebral compression fractures (Vertos II): an open-label randomized trial. Lancet. 2010;376:1085–92.
6. Wardlaw A, et al. Efficacy and safety of balloon kyphoplasty vs. non-surgical care for vertebral compression fracture (FREE): a randomized controlled trial. Lancet. 2009;373:1016.
7. Berenson A, et al. Balloon kyphoplasty versus non-surgical fracture management for treatment of painful vertebral body compression fractures in patients with cancer: a multicentre, randomized controlled trial. Lancet Oncol. 2011;12:225–35.
8. Edidin A, et al. Morbidity and mortality after vertebral fractures. Spine. 2015;40(15):1228–41.

Surgical Interventions for Pain

41

Robert J. Wilson II and Ginger E. Holt

Low Back Pain

Chronic low back pain is a common reason for hospital admission. The keys to determining if surgical treatment is indicated for hospitalized chronic low back pain patients are a thorough patient history, physical examination and judicious use of imaging studies.

The history should focus on determining the anatomic site, character, inciting factors, current treatment regimen, presence of neurologic deficits and past treatments for the pain. Whether the patient has any so-called "red flags" of back pain (Chap. 7) (Table 41.1) [1], is important as these may be the reason for admission for acute worsening of chronic pain and may necessitate more urgent intervention.

Table 41.1 Red flags of back pain	
	Older age
	History of trauma
	Prolonged corticosteroid use
	Fever
	Injection drug use
	Neurological deficit
	History of cancer

R. J. Wilson II
Department of Orthopaedics, Baptist MD Anderson Cancer Center, Jacksonville, FL, USA

G. E. Holt (✉)
Department of Orthopaedics, Vanderbilt University Medical Center, Nashville, TN, USA
e-mail: ginger.e.holt@vumc.org

© Springer Nature Switzerland AG 2022
D. A. Edwards et al. (eds.), *Hospitalized Chronic Pain Patient*,
https://doi.org/10.1007/978-3-031-08376-1_41

The physical examination should focus on strength testing of the major muscle groups of the upper and lower extremities as well as testing for sensation to pain, light touch and proprioception. Upper extremity neurologic examination is important to rule-out cervical or thoracic stenosis or myelopathy leading to lower extremity neurologic dysfunction. Reflex testing should be performed as well. Asking the patient to walk and perform tandem gait are useful tests as well to check for myelopathy. Rectal examination to evaluate rectal tone is recommended.

Imaging studies the low back in patients with chronic low back pain can cloud the clinical picture if not ordered for the correct indications [2]. Imaging studies, especially advanced imaging studies such as computed tomography (CT) or magnetic resonance imaging (MRI), will frequently show *radiographic* evidence of pathology in the lumbo-sacral spine, especially as patients age. However, correlating the radiographically evident pathology with the history and physical exam findings is paramount. If the radiographic findings do not correlate with patient symptoms and the physical exam, alternative explanations for the pain must be sought.

Antero- posterior (AP) and upright flexion and extension dynamic lateral plain lumbar spine radiographs are the recommended initial imaging study for patients hospitalized with chronic low back pain. The flexion and extension radiographs help identify dynamic instability in the lumbar spine consistent with spondylolisthesis ("slipped disc"). If there is a history of recent trauma, all imaging studies should be performed supine without dynamic views to abide by strict spine precautions. CT scans of the spine, in addition to or in lieu of, plain radiographs are the study of choice for diagnosis of vertebral fractures, especially in the cervical spine [3]. CT myelograms are helpful for evaluating spinal stenosis, epidural abscesses or hematoma, disc herniation or other causes of spinal compression in those patients who cannot undergo MRI scans or those with pre-existing spinal hardware.

The appropriate use of lumbar MRI and other advanced imaging studies in hospitalized chronic low back pain patients is essential and challenging [2]. Worsening of chronic low back pain alone, without associated signs or symptoms such as the "red flags", is not sufficient to justify ordering advanced imaging as often the clinical outcome is not changed by the study [2].

Surgery for chronic low back pain in hospitalized patients is one part of a myriad of treatment options. Any decision to proceed with surgical intervention should be made with expert input from a spine surgery specialist. A clinical practice guideline was published in 2009 which included interventional and surgical techniques for low back pain [4]. The grading system for the guidelines is listed as A (strong evidence/should recommend), B (fair evidence/reasonable to recommend), C (fair evidence/cannot recommend for or against), D (fair evidence/should *not* recommend), I (insufficient evidence/cannot recommend for or against) [4]. The treatment recommendations, indications and level of evidence for surgical treatments are summarized in Table 41.2.

Table 41.2 Summary of recommendations for surgical intervention for low back pain

Surgery	Clinical indication	Level of evidence	Recommendation grade
Fusion surgery	Non-radicular low back pain with common degenerative changes	Fair	B
Artificial disc replacement	Single-level degenerative disc disease	Fair	B (through 2 year), I (long-term outcomes)
Open discectomy or Microdiscectomy	Radiculopathy with prolapsed lumbar disc	Good	B
Laminectomy with or without fusion	Symptomatic spinal stenosis with or without degenerative spondylolisthesis	Good	B

Osteoarthritis/Rheumatoid Arthritis

Chronic pain from osteoarthritis (OA) or Rheumatoid Arthritis (RA) is common [5]. Patients may be hospitalized with intermittent flairs of significant joint pain in either condition. When these patients are admitted the history and physical exam should focus on ruling out alternative causes of joint pain. A recent history of trauma should increase the suspicion for a periarticular fracture. A recent febrile illness or current fevers should alert the clinician a superimposed joint infection may be present. A concurrent history of gout or other crystalline arthropathies should be elicited. Changes in pain regimen, or disease modifying agents in the case of RA, may cause an exacerbation of pain as well. If the patient has recently increased their activities, then a painful exacerbation of either arthritis type is possible. Furthermore, a stress fracture is also possible especially because OA and RA patients with chronic pain are likely older or possibly taking systemic corticosteroids and thus bone quality may be poor.

The physical exam should focus on identifying the joint(s) affected and the severity of the involvement. If the patient has lower extremity joint involvement the ability to walk should be ascertained. The location of the pain and whether it is reproduced with range of motion of adjacent joint(s) is essential. For example, it is often forgotten that medial groin pain is more indicative of hip joint pain that lateral thigh pain, which is more indicative of greater trochanteric bursitis. The presence of joint effusions should be evaluated. In addition, it is important to ask the patient if a specific joint is more swollen than usual, as both OA and RA patients are likely to have chronic joint effusions. The range of motion of affected joints should be examined. Pain with both active and passive range of motion in the presence of an increased effusion, erythema and warmth of a joint increases the suspicion of infection.

Imaging evaluation should almost always begin with AP and lateral plain radiographs of the affected joint(s). If a lower extremity joint is involved the plain radiographs should be taken with the patient weight bearing if possible. Weight bearing radiographs are superior to non-weight bearing radiographs for evaluating the joint space narrowing indicative of arthritis [6].

If occult fracture is suspected a CT or MRI scan of the affected bone and adjacent joint are recommended. If a peri-articular soft tissue mass, infection or intra-articular ligamentous or meniscal injury is suspected MRI of the joint is recommended. Bone scans can also detect occult fractures and bone infections however their usefulness is reduced in OA and RA as these conditions have increased tracer uptake in affected joints at baseline.

Laboratory work-up is primarily indicated to help differentiate between chronic OA or RA pain and septic arthritis or crystalline arthropathies. C-reactive protein (CRP) levels and erythrocyte sedimentation (ESR) levels should be drawn if there is suspicion of infection. If elevated, especially in a patient with joint swelling and fever, it should raise the concern for superimposed infection. CRP and ESR elevations in RA patients are likely not as sensitive or specific for infection but comparing current lab values to prior values if available can help determine if the values are elevated beyond the patient's baseline RA inflammation. If the history, exam, imaging and laboratory values are concerning for joint infection, aspiration of joint fluid is indicated. The typical synovial fluid aspiration results of OA, RA and septic arthritis are beyond the scope of this chapter. The joint aspiration and interpretation of the results should be performed with the assistance of a rheumatologist and/or orthopedic surgeon.

Surgery for debilitating chronic joint pain depends on the joint affected and the etiology and orthopaedic surgery consultation in recommended for the hospitalized chronic joint pain patient. If septic arthritis is present prompt irrigation and debridement of the affected joint is recommended. Common surgical options for chronic OA or RA include arthroplasty (joint replacement) and arthrodesis (joint fusion). For the shoulder, hip and knee, total joint arthroplasty is the mainstay of treatment and reliably reduces pain and increases function in both OA and RA patients [7, 8]. Arthrodesis of the shoulder, hip or knee is not recommended when arthroplasty is possible. For small joints of the hand, and foot and the ankle and wrist joints arthrodesis is commonly used as well. Total elbow replacement and total ankle replacement have more prominent roles in RA patients. The surgical options for chronic joint pain from OA or RA are reasonable to consider and of reliable benefit when patients are refractory to conservative options such as medication management, physical therapy, bracing and injections.

Cancer-Related Musculoskeletal Pain

Skeletal metastatic disease is a significant cause of chronic pain, loss of function and permanent disability [9]. The most common cancers causing bony metastatic disease are lung, breast, prostate, renal and thyroid carcinomas [10]. Multiple myeloma is another potential cause of chronic bone pain. Typically, this patient population has incurable, advanced stage cancer and thus complete resolution of pain and disability is unlikely. The essential goals of treatment for bony metastatic disease are: pain management, slowing or halting disease progression and preserving musculoskeletal function. A multidisciplinary team is therefore needed. Medical oncology, radiation oncology, orthopedic surgery, pain specialists, nutritionists and palliative care specialists all play essential roles in treating these patients.

There are two populations of skeletal metastatic disease patients to consider: those with known skeletal metastatic disease hospitalized with chronic pain and those who have chronic pain presenting with skeletal metastatic disease for the first time. The patient group with known metastatic disease is more straightforward and medical treatment of pain and radiation and/or surgical treatment can commence immediately. Consultation from pain specialists, orthopedic surgery, radiation oncology, medical oncology and palliative care should be sought as appropriate to help determine overall treatment course and the specific treatment for various skeletal sites of disease.

The patient who is hospitalized with a new lytic bone lesion with or without a personal cancer history is more challenging. The history should focus on the duration, location and character of the pain. Pain that is worse with weight bearing and better with laying or sitting down should raise suspicion for a pathologic fracture. Trivial injury mechanisms such as fracturing the femur while getting up from a chair should be considered a pathologic fracture due to malignancy until proven otherwise. The past medical history should focus on identifying any personal history of cancer, relevant occupational exposures, smoking history and constitutional symptoms such as fever, weight loss and anorexia. Questions about hematuria, hematochezia, hemoptysis and difficulty swallowing can help narrow down the possible primary cancer site. The results of recent mammograms, colonoscopies, urinalyses, chest radiographs and laboratory results such as prostate specific antigen (PSA) testing should be sought or inquired about in the history. Questions should also focus on identifying addition sites of pain as these may represent other sites of bony involvement.

The physical exam should focus on palpable of painful areas looking for bony and soft tissues masses including the spine. A breast exam should be performed to check for palpable masses. A prostate exam is recommended. The ability for the patient to ambulate should be evaluated.

Imaging work-up should begin with AP and lateral plain radiographs of the entire affected bone(s). More than one lesion may exist in the symptomatic bone thus imaging the entire bone is essential. Once plain radiographs identify a lesion concerning for bony metastatic disease further imaging and lab work-up is appropriate. Skeletal metastases usually cause bone destruction and cause the bone to have a "moth-eaten" appearance indicative of punctate areas of bony lysis [11]. Occasionally, especially in the case of prostate or breast carcinoma, the bone can be stimulated to make more bone by the tumor causing increased bone formation ("blastic metastases") [12]. It is important to note that not all lytic bone lesions are metastatic carcinoma. Primary bone sarcoma, benign bone tumors, infections and bone metabolic abnormalities can also have a similar appearance [13]. MRI and CT scans are indicated of the affected bone to evaluate associated soft tissue masses and help with surgical planning as indicated. They are not substitutes for plain radiographs.

Once a bone lesion is identified a specific imaging and lab work-up is indicated to help determine the origin of the cancer and complete staging. A CT of the chest, abdomen and pelvis with intravenous contrast and a whole-body bone scan are indicated. Labs should include a complete metabolic panel, PSA test in a male, and serum and urine protein electrophoresis to check for multiple myeloma. A study found that this diagnostic strategy for a patient presenting with a lytic bone lesion identified the primary site malignancy 85% of the time [14]. Positron emission tomography combined with triple CT scans are indicated for initial staging and surveillance of certain malignancies as well [15].

Once the staging is completed, the next step is a biopsy for tissue sampling of an appropriate lesion. Doing this after the staging work-up is recommended as the staging work-up may find a more easily accessible and thus safer lesion to biopsy. Orthopaedic surgery consultation is recommended to evaluate the need for biopsy and potentially palliative surgical intervention for the lesion(s). It is vitally important that the biopsy, even if percutaneous, and any potential surgery is carefully planned in concert with the surgical team to prevent mistakes in the execution of the biopsy [16]. There are a myriad of surgical options for chronic pain caused by skeletal metastases including fracture fixation, arthroplasty, arthrodesis and amputation. The discussion and indications of each is beyond the scope of this chapter. However, palliative surgery for painful skeletal metastases in concert with radiation and medical oncology typically decreases pain and increases or maintains patient function [17].

Summary
- Chronic low back pain alone is not sufficient justification for advance imaging work-up or surgical intervention. Surgery has efficacy in specific causes of chronic low back pain with the appropriate associated imaging and physical exam findings.
- Chronic joint pain in Osteoarthritis or Rheumatoid Arthritis responds well to arthroplasty or fusion of the affected joint when conservative options have been exhausted.
- Chronic pain from skeletal metastatic disease is debilitating and requires a multidisciplinary team to optimize patient care. Surgery is palliative and can decrease pain and maintain function.

References

1. Downie A, Williams CM, Henschke N, Hancock MJ, Ostelo RW, de Vet HC, Macaskill P, Irwig L, van Tulder MW, Koes BW, Maher CG. Red flags to screen for malignancy and fracture in patients with low back pain: systematic review. BMJ. 2013;347:7095.

2. Chou R, Fu R, Carrino JA, Deyo RA. Imaging strategies for low-back pain: systematic review and meta-analysis. Lancet. 2009;373(9662):463–72.
3. Parizel PM, Van der Zijden T, Gaudino S, Spaepen M, Voormolen MH, Venstermans C, De Belder F, van den Hauwe L, Van Goethem J. Trauma of the spine and spinal cord: imaging strategies. Eur Spine J. 2010;19(1):8–17.
4. Chou R, Loeser JD, Owens DK, Rosenquist RW, Atlas SJ, Baisden J, Carragee EJ, Grabois M, Murphy DR, Resnick DK, Stanos SP. Interventional therapies, surgery, and interdisciplinary rehabilitation for low back pain: an evidence-based clinical practice guideline from the American Pain Society. Spine. 2009;34(10):1066–77.
5. Johannes CB, Le TK, Zhou X, Johnston JA, Dworkin RH. The prevalence of chronic pain in United States adults: results of an internet-based survey. J Pain. 2010;11(11):1230–9.
6. Leach RE, Gregg T, Siber FJ. Weight-bearing radiography in osteoarthritis of the knee 1. Radiology. 1970;97(2):265–8.
7. Bruyère O, Ethgen O, Neuprez A, Zegels B, Gillet P, Huskin JP, Reginster JY. Health-related quality of life after total knee or hip replacement for osteoarthritis: a 7-year prospective study. Arch Orthop Trauma Surg. 2012;132(11):1583–7.
8. Lo IK, Litchfield RB, Griffin S, Faber K, Patterson SD, Kirkley A. Quality-of-life outcome following hemiarthroplasty or total shoulder arthroplasty in patients with osteoarthritis. J Bone Joint Surg Am. 2005;87(10):2178–85.
9. Cleeland CS. The measurement of pain from metastatic bone disease: capturing the patient's experience. Clin Cancer Res. 2006;12(20):6236–42.
10. Coleman RE. Clinical features of metastatic bone disease and risk of skeletal morbidity. Clin Cancer Res. 2006;12(20):6243.
11. Yarmenitis SD. Conventional radiology of bone and soft tissue tumors. In: Imaging in clinical oncology. Milan: Springer; 2014. p. 83–8.
12. Messiou C, Cook G. Imaging metastatic bone disease from carcinoma of the prostate. Br J Cancer. 2009;101(8):1225–32.
13. Miller TT. Bone tumors and tumorlike conditions: analysis with conventional radiography 1. Radiology. 2008;246(3):662–74.
14. Rougraff BT, Kneisl JS, Simon MA. Skeletal metastases of unknown origin. A prospective study of a diagnostic strategy. J Bone Joint Surg Am. 1993;75(9):1276–81.
15. Bar-Shalom R, Yefremov N, Guralnik L, Gaitini D, Frenkel A, Kuten A, Altman H, Keidar Z, Israel O. Clinical performance of PET/CT in evaluation of cancer: additional value for diagnostic imaging and patient management. J Nucl Med. 2003;44(8):1200–9.
16. Mankin HJ, Mankin CJ, Simon MA. The hazards of the biopsy, revisited. For the members of the Musculoskeletal Tumor Society. J Bone Joint Surg Am. 1996;78(5):656–3.
17. Wood TJ, Racano A, Yeung H, Farrokhyar F, Ghert M, Deheshi BM. Surgical management of bone metastases: quality of evidence and systematic review. Ann Surg Oncol. 2014;21(13):4081–9.

Part VI

Palliative Care

Opioid and Non-opioid Therapies in Palliative Care

42

Andrew Wooldridge, Stacy D. Tillman, and April Zehm

Non-opioid Therapies

One key benefit to the palliative care approach is interdisciplinary team-based care. This can be especially helpful in the vulnerable population with advanced or life-limiting illness and co-morbid chronic pain. Palliative care patients can experience "total pain" when physical pain combines with psychological, existential, and spiritual distress. Approaches such as social work therapy, chaplain counseling, and psychotherapy are essential in addressing the total pain that comes serious and life-threatening illness and can often help lessen pain medication requirements.

Non-pharmacological approaches should always be considered as a complement to pharmacological approaches. Though availability of some integrative services may vary, there is a growing body of literature to support these interventions, even in the acute setting, and we recommend to always review what may be available in your institution [1].

Significant attention is devoted to multimodal agents for the hospitalized chronic pain patient in other areas (Part IV Medication Treatments). However, special attention can be given to some agents when poor prognosis changes the risk/benefit equation. Specifically, one may be more accepting of the long-term side effect profile and more likely to recommend an agent if prognosis is so poor that long-term side effects are unlikely to manifest. Conversely, if an agent needs a long time to titrate up to reach full effect, then its efficacy may be diminished in a limited-prognosis situation.

A. Wooldridge · S. D. Tillman (✉)
Department of Medicine, Division of Palliative Care, Vanderbilt University Medical Center, Nashville, TN, USA
e-mail: stacy.d.tillman@vumc.org

A. Zehm
Division of Geriatric and Palliative Medicine, Clinical Cancer Center, Medical College of Wisconsin, Milwaukee, WI, USA
e-mail: azehm@mcw.edu

© Springer Nature Switzerland AG 2022
D. A. Edwards et al. (eds.), *Hospitalized Chronic Pain Patient*,
https://doi.org/10.1007/978-3-031-08376-1_42

NSAIDs

NSAIDs can be highly efficacious in treating inflammatory pain. However, their use is often limited by the risk of side effects, most notably kidney failure or gastritis and peptic ulcer disease. While we always consider risk/benefit ratio carefully in palliative care and often use medications more willingly than other disciplines, we do recognize that our patient population is at higher risk of dehydration, anorexia and polypharmacy, which could cause renal failure or gastritis that would then be exacerbated using NSAIDs. One study showed that in the week before death, 60% of patients had impaired kidney function that was previously unknown, and 19% had severe renal failure. Many of these patients were on Morphine or NSAIDs [2]. This poses the risk of accumulation of drugs and potential toxicity, which could negatively affect quality of life as a patient is dying. Therefore, careful consideration should be taken when prescribing NSAIDs for longer periods, even in patients with limited prognoses.

Corticosteroids

Concern for adverse effects from long-term use of glucocorticoids generally prohibits the use of these as adjuvant therapy in patients with chronic pain. However, in patients with limited life expectancy the potential benefits of steroids may outweigh the risks of side effects. In addition to their analgesic effects, steroids have beneficial effects on appetite, fatigue, depressed mood and nausea, which often contribute to poor quality of life in those with advanced disease [3].

Dexamethasone is typically the steroid of choice given its high potency, low mineralocorticoid effects (and thus less fluid retention), long half-life allowing for once daily dosing, low cost, and availability of oral and parenteral formulations [2, 3].

Short term adverse effects of steroids include immunosuppression (often manifested as oral thrush), hyperglycemia, edema, and psychological changes (insomnia, agitation, delirium). Steroids should be used with caution in patients who are already at risk for these complications, such as those with immunosuppression from chemotherapy, underlying diabetes or congestive heart failure, or delirium. Caution should be taken if using steroids in conjunction with NSAIDs as this increases the risk of gastric bleeding; prophylactic gastric protectants should be prescribed in all of these patients. Lastly, in the era of immunotherapeutics in oncology, steroids should be avoided in a patient on an immunotherapy unless discussed with the patient's oncologist.

Given the risk of adverse effects increases with the dose of the drug and the duration of use, care should be taken to choose the lowest effective dose. There is limited data to guide dexamethasone dosing in palliative patients, and a wide range is often seen in clinical practice. We suggest a starting dose of dexamethasone 2–8 mg daily or in divided BID doses (with the second dose of the day given around 2 pm to avoid nocturnal side effects).

Often when a terminally ill patient is started on steroids the intention is to continue until the patient dies if they are providing benefit. However, if steroids do not improve the patient's symptoms or cause adverse effects, they should be discontinued. If steroids have been given for less than three weeks, suppression of the HPA axis is rare and steroids can be stopped without a taper. Steroids should be reduced gradually if the patient has been taking for longer than 3 weeks. In patients who may be on moderate to high doses steroids for more than a couple of weeks, pneumocystis carinii pneumonia (PCP) prophylaxis should be considered.

Neuropathic Agents

Neuropathic agents such as gabapentin, pregabalin, tricyclic antidepressants (TCAs), and duloxetine can be helpful in the palliative care setting. Choice of a neuropathic agent should be tailored to the patient's medical issues and co-morbidities. For example, a TCA should be avoided in a frail elderly patient with a history of falls and urinary retention, but could be very helpful in a young patient with neuropathic pain, depression, and insomnia. As noted above, it is important to consider that it may take weeks for these agents to be titrated to an effective dose, and patients with a short prognosis may not have the luxury of waiting for these agents to take effect.

Cannabinoids

Numerous studies have demonstrated benefit of cannabinoids in treating various types of chronic pain, most notably neuropathic pain [1]. A 2015 meta-analysis looking at the use of cannabinoids for various medical disorders showed smoked THC and nabiximols improved chronic neuropathic or cancer pain compared with placebo controls [1]. Nabiximols, a 1:1 mixture of THC and cannabidiol as an oromucosal spray, have been shown to be an effective and safe adjunct in treating opioid-refractory cancer pain [1]. In animal models, cannabinoids and opioids have been shown to have synergistic analgesic effects.

These studies indicate a potential for cannabinoid drugs to be used as adjuvant pain medications, especially in patients with difficult, refractory pain or severe neuropathy. This agent is not currently FDA-approved but is undergoing Phase III trials for use for pain in the USA. It is already available in other countries.

Opioid Therapies

These agents are described in detail elsewhere, see Part IV Medication Treatments for details. The focus of this section will be how these principles apply specifically to the palliative care setting.

Titration and Rotation

As noted, this topic is covered in-depth elsewhere in Part IV Medication Treatments. Although we try to limit use of these agents in chronic pain syndrome, we may be more liberal with our titration in patients with a comorbid diagnosis that benefits from palliative care involvement, such as those with acute and progressive pain sources associated with a poor prognosis.

Opioid Side Effects

Constipation
Opioid-induced constipation (OIC) can occur with any opioids at any dose, and patients do not develop tolerance to this over time. Palliative care patients usually have significant disease burden leading to numerous risk factors for constipation, including poor oral intake, immobility, electrolyte abnormalities, and use of offending drugs such as anticholinergics and diuretics. Consider initiation of Senna 2–8 tabs/day in divided doses and polyethylene glycol 17 g daily to twice a day as an initial strategy for OIC [4]. If ineffective, either bisacodyl 5–15 mg po daily or lactulose 30–60 ml daily can be added. If patients do not have a bowel movement after 3–4 days, they may need either a suppository or enema, and impaction may need to be ruled out if a patient is not neutropenic or thrombocytopenia. Of note, data suggests that, despite widespread use, docusate is no more effective than senna and should no longer be routinely used.

Nausea and Vomiting
General management of this and explanation of the phenomenon is covered elsewhere, in Part IV Medication Treatments.

Sedation/Delirium
Opiates can cause delirium even at low doses, but this effect is usually reversible. If suspected, this should be managed with dose reduction or opioid rotation [5]. Delirium is common at the end of life and can be compounded by numerous factors seen in hospitalized patients. Therefore, the cause of delirium in advanced disease is likely multifactorial and should be managed with treatment of any reversible causes, environmental strategies, and pharmacologic intervention if necessary for agitated, hyperactive delirium.

These side effects can be disconcerting for patients and family members as they can prohibit communication and valuable time with loved ones in patients with limited prognoses. We counsel family (and sometimes can even pre-counsel with patient) that using these agents with the goal of comfort carries these risks, and we always work to balance relief of pain and suffering with quality time with families.

When opiates are titrated appropriately, even in patients with advanced disease or who are actively dying, analgesia can be achieved prior to causing unintended sedation [5]. We strongly recommend reviewing the extensive literature and evidence showing that appropriate use and titration of opioid agents does not hasten death so that we can avoid propagating the myth of hastened death to patients and families as well as other providers.

References

1. Abrams DI. Integrating cannabis into clinical cancer care. Curr Oncol. 2016;23(2):S8–S14.
2. Hanks G. Oxford textbook palliative medicine. 4th ed. Oxford: Oxford University Press; 2011. p. 712–3.
3. Leppert W, Buss T. The role of corticosteroids in the treatment of pain in cancer patients. Curr Pain Headache Rep. 2012;16(4):307–13.
4. Swarm RA, et al. Adult cancer pain, version 3.2019, NCCN clinical practice guidelines in oncology. J Natl Compr Cancer Netw. 2019;17(8):977–1007.
5. Lawlor PG, Gagnon B, Mancini IL, Pereira JL, Hanson J, Suarez-Almazor ME, Bruera ED. Occurrence, causes, and outcome of delirium in patients with advanced cancer: a prospective study. Arch Intern Med. 2000;160(6):786–94.

Crisis Management and Refractory Pain

43

Mihir M. Kamdar, April Zehm,
and Bethany-Rose Daubman

Assessment of a Patient in a Pain Crisis

All patients should receive a careful history and physical examination, including a detailed pain assessment (Table 43.1). Assess psychological and spiritual symptoms and the patient's understanding of the cause or meaning of their pain, as anxiety, depression, delirium, and existential suffering can impact the pain experience and its management [3].

Additional diagnostic workup should be individualized, and depends on the patient's underlying disease, prognosis, preferences and goals of care. If the pain is an abrupt change in clinical status, the evaluation may include diagnostic procedures, especially if results will lead to potentially effective treatments that would improve quality of life. However, if the burdens or risks of additional diagnostic testing outweigh potential benefits within the context of the patient's illness trajectory, further diagnostics may not be indicated. The management plan and rationale should be clearly documented, especially if shared decision-making leads to a decision to forego additional workup and focus on comfort.

M. M. Kamdar
Division of Palliative Care, Massachusetts General Hospital, Harvard University, Boston, MA, USA

Division of Anesthesia Pain Medicine, Massachusetts General Hospital, Harvard University, Boston, MA, USA
e-mail: mmkamdar@mgh.harvard.edu

A. Zehm
Division of Geriatric and Palliative Medicine, Department of Medicine, Medical College of Wisconsin, Milwaukee, WI, USA
e-mail: azehm@mcw.edu

B.-R. Daubman (✉)
Division of Palliative Care and Geriatrics, Department of Medicine, Massachusetts General Hospital, Harvard University, Boston, MA, USA
e-mail: bdaubman@mgh.harvard.edu

© Springer Nature Switzerland AG 2022
D. A. Edwards et al. (eds.), *Hospitalized Chronic Pain Patient*,
https://doi.org/10.1007/978-3-031-08376-1_43

Table 43.1 Assessment of a patient in a pain crisis [1, 2]

- Believe the patient's complaint of pain
- Take a careful pain history and contextualize it within the patient's illness history
- Evaluate for contributing or confounding psychological symptoms (delirium, anxiety, existential crisis, etc.) and history of substance use disorder
- Perform a careful medical and neurologic examination
- Define the goals of the pain intervention
- Individualize diagnostic and therapeutic strategies that are congruent with goals of care
- Order appropriate diagnostic studies swiftly, depending on benefit-burden ratio
- Treat the pain while concomitantly determining etiology of the pain
- Provide continual monitoring and support of the patient and family until the crisis is controlled
- Reassess the patient's response to therapy on an ongoing basis, documenting meticulously
- Involve the interdisciplinary team to assist with psychosocial support and nonpharmacologic means of pain management

Management of a Pain Crisis

While additional diagnostics are being considered, pain management should begin immediately as it can be time and labor-intensive. Pain intensity, degree of relief, and adverse effects of therapy should be closely monitored until the pain crisis has resolved. Effective communication is critical for patient and family, particularly regarding the management plan and coping techniques. Reassure the patient that you will remain present until the crisis is resolved.

Opioids

Route

Patients with severe pain should receive rapid and aggressive titration of an opioid analgesic, possibly with the addition of non-opioid adjuvants. Parenteral administration (intravenous (IV) or subcutaneous (SC) if IV access is unavailable) is the preferred route of opioid delivery during a pain crisis.

Starting Doses

For opioid-naive patients, 2–4 mg IV morphine or an equianalgesic dose of a different opioid is a reasonable starting dose. For opioid-tolerant patients, convert the patient's usual oral rescue dose to an IV equivalent using relative potency tables, and administer 100–150% of this dose. Alternatively, it is reasonable to administer the IV equivalent of 10–15% of the patient's total daily opioid requirement (calculated by summing all long and short-acting opioids in a 24-h period).

Titrate Based on Response

Once an appropriate opioid dose has been selected, the dose should be rapidly titrated until the patient either has relief of pain or intolerable side effects develop. Parenteral opioids can be administered to the patient every 15–30 min as needed, a time interval that is based on the approximate time to peak analgesic effect. Further management depends on the clinical response.

Non-opioid Adjuvant Medications

Non-opioid adjuvant or co-analgesic medications should be considered early in a pain crisis management strategy [4]. Adjuvant drugs can enhance the effects of opioids, exert independent analgesic effects for certain types of pain, and counteract opioid side effects, widening the therapeutic window [2]. Parenteral non-steroidal anti-inflammatory medications such as ketorolac can be markedly helpful, as they provide equianalgesic pain relief to morphine but spare opioid side effects, however risks of gastrointestinal bleeding, thrombocytopenia, and kidney injury must be considered [5]. Steroids may be helpful for a subset of patients, particularly if pain is felt to be due to tumor infiltration causing inflammation and edema [6]. Ketamine has been shown to be a potent analgesic and may potentiate opioid analgesia, reduce pain, and allow significant dose reductions of other analgesics. Table 43.2 illustrates parenteral adjuvants that can be used in a pain crisis.

Refractory Pain

While opioid rotation can often alleviate dose-limiting side effects, sedation can be a challenging side effect to circumvent when treating cancer pain. Within a larger goals of care framework, it can be helpful to ask the patient about the acceptability of sedation if the only way to adequately control pain, particularly if there is clinical concern about a narrow therapeutic window. For patients with refractory pain or intolerable side effects, neuraxial (epidural or intrathecal) drug delivery, interventional procedures or surgical techniques to control pain should be considered.

Sometimes it is impossible to control pain despite maximal medical and interventional therapies. In these instances, proportionate palliative sedation may be considered as a tool of last resort. This involves the use of progressively higher levels of sedation (potentially to the level of unconsciousness) to help relieve otherwise intractable suffering. If palliative sedation is being considered, it is imperative to have experts in palliative care and ethics involved to ensure all other therapeutic options have been considered and the circumstances warrant this intervention.

Table 43.2 Parenteral adjuvant co-analgesics for use in pain crisis management

Drugs	Dosing	Indications	Notes
Non-steroidal anti-inflammatories • Ketorolac	15–30 mg initially, then 15–30 mg Q6H PRN for up to 5 days	Neuropathic pain Visceral pain Bone pain Inflammatory pain Soft tissue infiltration Hepatomegaly	Equianalgesic to morphine Caution GI effects Renal toxicity may precipitate ARF in dehydrated patients; consider co-hydration
Corticosteroids • Dexamethasone	Varies If spinal cord compression, 10 mg load followed by 16 mg/day in divided doses For bone pain, 2–16 mg/day in divided doses, then taper	Bone metastasis Elevated intracranial pressure Soft tissue infiltration Spinal/nerve compression Hepatomegaly	Risk of GI bleeding, insomnia, hyperglycemia, delirium, psychosis, etc.
Ketamine	0.1–0.5 mg/kg loading dose followed by 1.65–5 mcg/kg/min, titrating up every 4–6 h as needed For higher doses, consider ICU monitoring	Intractable pain Neuropathic pain Opioid side effects Opioid-induced hyperalgesia	Risk of dissociative effects, hallucinations, cardiovascular effects (arrhythmias, brady/tachycardia, hypo/hypertension)
Lidocaine	1 mg/kg loading dose followed by 0.5–2 mg/kg/h up to 4 mg/kg/h	Intractable pain Neuropathic pain	Risk of vertigo, blood pressure and heart rate changes, altered mental status, seizures

Assessing for Psychological Distress

Patients with serious illness may experience intractable pain, especially when complicated by psychological distress. Psychological distress may be defined as a patient's inner state of suffering resulting from physical, psychological, social, spiritual, and/or practical issues. Though patients experience both physical and psychological pain, standard medical treatments usually target only the physical pain, however, psychological factors can significantly impede pain management. Oftentimes, patients will somatize their feelings, resulting in amplified pain expression, which may be difficult to control without addressing the psychological basis behind it. In turn, lack of care for psychosocial distress can increase pain severity and result in escalation of pharmacological pain treatments.

A multi-dimensional approach to intractable pain is the recommended pathway. Exploring a patient's pain experience through physical, psychological, social, and spiritual lenses provides a more comprehensive evaluation, and may lead to treatment of co-morbid depression or anxiety, or attention to particular social or spiritual distresses. An interdisciplinary team involving social workers, psychologists, and chaplains may also support patients experiencing psychological distress. Interventions may include pharmacological management of depression and anxiety, supportive counseling, and demonstration of relaxation techniques such as guided imagery and meditation.

References

1. Moryl N, Coyle N, Foley K. Managing an acute pain crisis in a patient with advanced cancer: "this is as much of a crisis as a code". JAMA. 2008;299(12):1457–67.
2. Foley K. Management of cancer pain. In: DeVita V, Hellman S, Rosenberg S, editors. Cancer principles and practice of oncology. 7th ed. Philadelphia: Lippincott Williams & Wilkins; 2005. p. 2615–49.
3. Wilson K, et al. Depression and anxiety disorders in palliative cancer care. J Pain Symptom Manag. 2007;33(2):118–29.
4. McNicol E, et al. Management of opioid side effects in cancer-related and chronic non-cancer pain: a systematic review. J Pain. 2003;4(5):231–56.
5. Mercadante S, Giarratano A. The long and winding road of non-steroidal ant inflammatory drugs and paracetamol in cancer pain management: a critical review. Crit Rev Oncol Hematol. 2013;87(2):140–5.
6. Paulsen O, Klepstad P, Rosland J, Aass N, Albert E, Fayers P, Kaasa S. Efficacy of methylprednisolone on pain, fatigue, and appetite loss in patients with advanced cancer using opioids: a randomized, placebo-controlled, double-blind trial. J Clin Oncol. 2014;32(29):3221–8.

Part VII

Discharge

Transition to Outpatient Care and Readmissions

44

Katheryne Lawson, David A. Edwards, and Andrew J. B. Pisansky

Transition to Outpatient Care of the Surgical Patient

No clear guidelines exist for managing postoperative pain as patients leave the hospital to recover as outpatients, especially for those with chronic pain already on a pain medication regimen [1]. However, it can take a comprehensive team including but not limited to chronic pain specialists, nurse practitioners, psychologists, physiotherapists with expertise in acupuncture and myofascial release, nursing staff, and patient-care coordinators to adequately care for these complex patients [2]. Without this team approach, patients with chronic pain taking opioids may end up leaving the hospital with a 100–300% increase in opioid medication dose from their baseline use after a major surgery and may not have an appropriate weaning plan for this dose increase to reflect their decreasing post-surgical pain as the body heals [1]. Frankly, even opioid-naïve patients are at risk for continued opioid use postoperatively as one study demonstrated that opioid-naïve patients who received a prescription for opioids within a week of low risk surgery had a 7.7% chance of continued opioid use 1 year later [3]. Completing a basic checklist for these patients can increase odds of a smooth transition from inpatient to outpatient management of acute on chronic pain and ultimately decrease readmissions, decrease pain-related

K. Lawson
Department of Anesthesiology, Royal Children's Hospital Melbourne, Parkville, VIC, Australia

D. A. Edwards (✉)
Departments of Anesthesiology and Neurological Surgery, Vanderbilt University Medical Center, Nashville, TN, USA
e-mail: david.a.edwards@vumc.org

A. J. B. Pisansky
Department of Anesthesiology, Vanderbilt University Medical Center, Nashville, TN, USA
e-mail: andrew.pisansky@vumc.org

© Springer Nature Switzerland AG 2022
D. A. Edwards et al. (eds.), *Hospitalized Chronic Pain Patient*,
https://doi.org/10.1007/978-3-031-08376-1_44

Table 44.1 To do list for discharge of patients with chronic pain

• Identify "at risk" patients
• Encourage and initiate preventative strategies and psychological intervention, as able
• Medication reconciliation
• Determine an appropriate opioid-sparing multimodal medication regimen
• Contact patient pharmacy
• Create a pain and opioid medication tapering schedule for discharge
• Schedule regular and early follow-up
• Provide patient with discharge instructions, including contact information of surgical and pain
  management teams
• Contact the patient's pain management physician and primary care physician to update them
  on inpatient status and/or medication changes
• Involve psychologist and physiotherapist colleagues at follow-up for alternative methods of
  pain control and to encourage continued pain and opioid medication taper

interference in relation to mobility, mood, and ability to work, and improve patient satisfaction (Table 44.1). Patients at significant risk for prolonged opioid use must first be identified so said patients can be targeted. Risk factors for prolonged opioid use include younger age, lower income, preoperative negative affective states including posttraumatic stress disorder symptoms, depression, anxiety, and pain catastrophizing, comorbidities, such as diabetes and heart failure, the presence of perioperative pain, and perioperative opioid, benzodiazepine, and antidepressant use [1, 2]. After identifying the "at risk" population whether at a preoperative appointment or prior to a scheduled procedure, preventative pharmacological strategies, prehabilitation, mindfulness, cognitive behavioral therapy, and yoga can be addressed and encouraged, as able, as a means to positively impact a patient's postoperative recovery [1]. One day psychoeducational workshops and pain optimization can empower patients preoperatively and postoperatively, with the goal of decreasing chronic postsurgical pain [1, 2]. The goals of psychological intervention prior to surgery are to assist patients in the development of personalized pain management plans, address distress and associated mental health issues that have the potential to amplify pain and increase opioid use, and support the ultimate weaning of opioid medications and return to baseline functionality [2].

Upon presentation for surgery, a medication reconciliation should be performed to make sure the patient's baseline medical problems and pain are treated effectively during the patient's inpatient stay. During this process, a patient's baseline morphine equivalents per day can be calculated for reference during the hospitalization.

Postoperatively, these patient's chronic pain in addition to their acute neuropathic, postsurgical pain should be effectively treated to the patient's satisfaction using an opioid-sparing multimodal medication regimen [2]. In a study done over a decade ago, Hayes et al. demonstrated that those who experience acute neuropathic pain were at risk of experiencing ongoing pain with 78% experiencing continued pain at 6 months and 56% experiencing continued pain at 12 months after surgery [4]. At this point, communication between the surgical team, pain management team, patient, and caregiver is of utmost importance to tailor pain medication regimens based on the expected trajectory of pain from the specific procedure performed. When making each patient's pain medication regimen, consideration of the patient's baseline regimen and morphine equivalents per day should be kept in mind to ensure that the patient's baseline needs are being met and that the regimen will not precipitate withdrawal. However, it should also be considered that the procedure performed might reduce the patient's baseline pain and that a patient's pain medication needs may ultimately be reduced after recovering from surgery.

Once the patient stabilizes and trends toward becoming medically and surgically appropriate for discharge, a member of the care team should meet with the patient and caregiver to determine a structured needs assessment [5]. Intravenous medications should be transitioned to medications by mouth or per tube, allowing time to reevaluate the patient's pain on this new regimen. If adequate by mouth or per tube medications are not available for a specific patient and they must be continued on an intravenous pain medication after discharge, the necessary coordination and referrals need to occur to ensure access to medication during transport, as well as at the destination [6]. Moreover, pharmacies need to be contacted to ensure such medications are available near the patient's destination and that they are cost effective for that patient [6]. At discharge, a comprehensive discharge plan should be enacted that includes patient and caregiver education with patient-centered discharge instructions, especially if new medications have been started or post-discharge services have been arranged [5]. It must be recognized that patient's caregivers and families have little or no training on how to care for the patient and his or her new pain [6]. A family meeting may be a useful method of consolidating this information [6]. Patients should be provided with a simple, easily readable pain medication and opioid weaning schedule, created in concert with the surgical team, that is based on expected postoperative pain and recovery from that patient's surgery (Table 44.2).

"At risk" patients and their caregivers should also have contact numbers or access to alternative electronic or mobile messaging system to allow questions pertaining to both surgical issues and pain in the postoperative period to be answered 24 h/day [2, 6]. Upon discharge, the primary inpatient care team and the inpatient pain management team, if not one in the same, should contact the patient's outpatient pain management physician and primary care physician to update them on the patient's hospitalization and/or medication changes [6].

One of the largest gaps in postsurgical care is the length of time between discharge and postsurgical follow up visits [1]. Approximately 10–20% of postsurgical patients are discharged without appropriate pain specialist follow-up to manage their complex postsurgical pain and to appropriately monitor the weaning of opioid medications [1]. Moreover, general practitioners may struggle with complex postsurgical pain patients because of lack of expertise and/or comfort in weaning patients from opioids, and patients aren't referred to chronic pain centers and specialists until 12–18 months after the pain has become chronic [1, 7]. This population should have their first follow-up phone call within 3 days of discharge and their first follow-up appointment in 2–3 weeks or sooner for those who need urgent care [1, 2]. The purpose of this first follow-up appointment is to assess patient progress and develop a plan for pain management and weaning from opioid medications [2]. At this visit, the patient is assessed for opioid addiction risk and a psychologist can be involved for those who are high-dose opioid users, who have a history of mental health problems, and who report significant distress and pain [2]. They can also be offered physiotherapy and/or acupuncture to restore function and attempt to relieve

Table 44.2 Expected course of pain from orthopedic surgery

Type of surgery: orthopedic procedure for fracture in the lower extremity		
With hardware		
Postoperative timing	What's expected?	Expected maximum dosage of pain medication above baseline
1–4 days	Postoperative pain at its maximum level	Opioid pain medication every 4 h as needed to control pain
5 days	Postoperative pain declining	Opioid pain medication every 12–24 h as needed to control pain
1 week	Postoperative pain continuing to decline	No opioid pain medication above baseline, multimodal pain medication regimen as prescribed and needed
6 weeks	Bone is nearly finished healing; physical therapy has started	No opioid pain medication above baseline, multimodal pain medication regimen as prescribed and needed
2–3 months	Return to baseline functioning	No opioid pain medication above baseline
Without hardware		
Postoperative timing	What's expected?	Expected maximum dosage of pain medication above baseline
1–4 days	Postoperative pain at its maximum level	Opioid pain medication every 4 h as needed to control pain
5 days	Postoperative pain declining	Opioid pain medication every 12 h as needed to control pain
1 week	Postoperative pain continuing to decline	Opioid pain medication every 24 h as needed to control pain
6 weeks	Bone is nearly finished healing; physical therapy has started	No opioid pain medication above baseline, multimodal pain medication regimen as prescribed and needed
4–6 months	Return to baseline functioning	No opioid pain medication above baseline

Note that weaning schedule above is simply an example and not based on data

pain [2]. The goal is to have patients back to their baseline functional status and medication usage within 6 weeks to 6 months after discharge, depending on the surgery.

Transition to Outpatient Care of the Medical Patient

The transition to outpatient care of a patient with chronic pain hospitalized for a medical reason embodies many of the same elements as in the transition to outpatient care of the surgical patient. It includes such things as communication between the patient, caregiver, pain management team, and primary inpatient care team to discuss diagnoses and prognoses, as well as what is to be expected based on the inpatient findings. It also can involve a team approach, should include a medication reconciliation, and requires timely follow-up after discharge. In essence, the "To Do" list in Table 44.1 is essentially the same with a few minor tweaks. A key difference between the transitions of these two types of patients is that in the case of a medical patient with chronic pain, the patient's pain level may not change significantly as a result of the disease process for which they are hospitalized. For example, a patient hospitalized for a COPD exacerbation may not have a significant increase in their overall pain relative to a patient hospitalized for a large spinal fusion. Alternatively, while surgical pain is expected to improve over time, chronic pain because of a medical process, such as cancer, may be expected to worsen over time and may require an escalating pain management plan. This may lead to inadequate pain management at home and subsequent readmissions if an appropriate support system is not in place.

Special Considerations: Use of Controlled Substances

If an inpatient is taking a controlled substance, such as methadone or suboxone, and is being prescribed this controlled substance from a specific clinic, the patient either needs to be continued on this medication according to their clinic's set schedule or the patient needs to be transitioned back to their clinic's set schedule prior to discharge. If a patient is taking suboxone, it can be discontinued while inpatient to effectively manage pain, but should be restarted when the patient has been weaned to minimal doses of oral opioid. The first dose of suboxone should occur once the patient is beginning to experience pain and would normally take a dose of oral opioid. Once suboxone has been restarted, oral opioids can be discontinued, based on home regimen. Failure to restart a patient's home controlled substance regimen may cause the patient to be discharged from that clinic because of medication nonadherence and or medication discrepancies. The patient's controlled substance clinic should be contacted while the patient is hospitalized to obtain more information about that patient's medication schedule, to alert the clinic that the patient is inpatient, and to assist in planning the patient's overall care [6].

Special Considerations: Caregiver and Family Support

Pain management in the home is a family experience, as the care provided to the patient effects the family system [6]. A system of ongoing monitoring and support for the patient and family should be in place to ensure the effectiveness of pain relief measures and early identification of caregiver burden and unmet needs [6]. Studies have reported an inverse relationship between the health and function of the cancer patient and the amount of caregiver burden with caregiver strain, depression and anxiety, resulting in poor outcomes for both the patient and caregiver [6]. Overall, caregivers are at higher risk of depression and heart disease and experience higher mortality rates [5]. Patient and caregiver fears of addiction and unfamiliarity with some of these medications can lead to under-reporting of pain and undermedication, as well as overtreatment of pain [6]. In one study, though patients and families reported parallel perception of a patient's cancer pain, family members consistently assessed the patient's level of pain somewhat higher than the patient [6]. Thus, education about the pain medications to be handled, medication side effects, and overdose is very important as caregivers' lack of knowledge about pain medications coupled with observing pain and suffering in a loved one and the overwhelming feeling of responsibility can contribute to significant caregiver and family distress [6]. Thus, while patient care is the priority, it is also imperative to provide the necessary support for the caregiver when a patient is discharged from the hospital, so a patient can be satisfactorily cared for in the outpatient setting and not be quickly readmitted.

References

1. Clarke H. Transitional pain medicine: novel pharmacological treatments for the management of moderate to severe postsurgical pain. Expert Rev Clin Pharmacol. 2016;9(3):345–9.
2. Katz J, Weinrib A, Fashler S, et al. The Toronto General Hospital transitional pain service: development and implementation of a multidisciplinary program to prevent chronic postsurgical pain. J Pain Res. 2015;8:695–702.
3. Alam A. Long-term analgesic use after low-risk surgery. Arch Intern Med. 2012;172(5):425.
4. Hayes C, Browne S, Lantry G, Burstal R. Neuropathic pain in the acute pain service: a prospective survey. Acute Pain. 2002;4(3):45–8.
5. Kripalani S, Theobald CN, Anctil B, Vasilevskis EE. Reducing hospital readmission rates: current strategies and future directions. Annu Rev Med. 2014;65(1):471–85.
6. Benzon HT, Rathmell JP, Wu CL, Turk DC, Argoff CE, Hurley RW. Practical management of pain. 5th ed. Philadelphia: Elsevier; 2014. p. 1040–8.
7. Huang A, Azam A, Segal S, et al. Chronic postsurgical pain and persistent opioid use following surgery: the need for a transitional pain service. Pain Manage. 2016;6(5):435–43.

Opioid Tapering for Acute on Chronic Non-cancer Pain

Arun Ganesh and Thomas E. Buchheit

Why Taper Opioids for Patients with Acute on Chronic Non-cancer Pain?

When patients on chronic opioid therapy are hospitalized with acute pain, ideally the use of non-opioid analgesics and neuraxial/regional anesthesia techniques (e.g., epidural and peripheral nerve blocks) can be used solely for treatment. However, the magnitude of acute pain in these patients is often high secondary to opioid tolerance and opioid induced hyperalgesia [1, 2]. Thus, escalation of the baseline opioid regimen or supplementation with parenteral opioids is frequently needed to treat their acute pain [3–6]. The 2016 Centers for Disease Control Guideline for Prescribing Opioids for Chronic Pain states that "benefits of high-dose opioids for chronic pain are not established" and that the "risks for serious harm related to opioid therapy increase at high opioid dosage." Patients on higher doses are at greater risk of motor vehicle injuries, overdose, and developing opioid use disorder (OUD), and the risks appear higher if patients are on >50 morphine milligram equivalents (MME) [7]. Additionally, risks of chronic opioid therapy develop at higher doses, including worsening constipation, hypogonadism, urinary retention, osteoporosis, and opioid induced hyperalgesia (OIH) [1, 7]. Thus, clinicians should try to minimize opioid dose escalation during acute pain episodes and should taper doses to baseline levels once acute pain subsides.

A. Ganesh (✉) · T. E. Buchheit
Department of Anesthesiology, Duke University School of Medicine, Durham, NC, USA
e-mail: arun.ganesh2@duke.edu; thomas.buchheit@duke.edu

© Springer Nature Switzerland AG 2022
D. A. Edwards et al. (eds.), *Hospitalized Chronic Pain Patient*,
https://doi.org/10.1007/978-3-031-08376-1_45

When to Taper Opioids for Acute on Chronic Non-cancer Pain

The duration of acute pain for patients on chronic opioid therapy is often longer compared to patients not on chronic opioid therapy [4]. It is generally not practical or cost-efficient to keep these patients hospitalized until acute pain completely resolves. Once acute pain has been controlled to acceptable levels without parenteral opioids, patients should be discharged on the oral opioid regimen that controlled their pain while inpatient (Table 45.1). Opioids should then be tapered as an outpatient to pre-admission levels as the acute pain further resolves (Table 45.1). This requires frequent follow up with patients in the weeks and months following

Table 45.1 Recommendations for tapering opioids in opioid dependent patients with acute on chronic non-cancer pain

Expected duration of acute pain	Examples	Goals of opioid tapering	Speed of opioid tapering
Short (<2 weeks)	• Laparoscopic surgeries • Skin lacerations • Acute pancreatitis • Renal colic	1. Minimize escalation of pre-admission opioid regimen while inpatient 2. Discharge patient on oral opioid regimen that controlled his/her pain while inpatient 3. Taper opioids to pre-admission levels as an outpatient as acute pain resolves	As acute pain resolves, taper additional opioid dose by 50% each week until patient is back to pre-admission opioid levels[a]
Long (>2 weeks)	• Orthopedic surgeries • Open abdominal surgeries • Rib fractures • major trauma	Same as above	As acute pain resolves, taper additional opioid dose by 25–33% every 1–2 weeks until patient is back to pre-admission opioid levels[b]

[a] Example: A patient on oxycodone 10 mg QID for chronic back pain is admitted for acute pancreatitis. He is acutely treated with IV opioids while NPO, and then successfully transitioned to oxycodone 20 mg QID on hospital day 3 when he is discharged. One week after discharge his abdominal pain is resolved and his opioids are tapered back to his baseline regimen of 10 mg QID
[b] Example: A patient on Morphine IR 30 mg TID for chronic neck pain presents for an open Whipple surgery. On post-op day 5 she is successfully transitioned from a continuous epidural infusion and IV opioids to PO Morphine IR 60 mg TID, and then discharged on post-op day 6 with this regimen. Two weeks after discharge, her incision pain has improved and she is tapered to Morphine IR 45 mg TID. Two weeks later she notes that her incision pain has completely resolved, and she is tapered to her baseline regimen of 30 mg TID

discharge from the hospital. The speed of the taper should be based on the expected duration of acute pain, with faster tapers for pain of shorter duration (Table 45.1).

We do not advise patients on chronic opioids be tapered below their baseline opioid regimen while admitted for acute pain. Doing so would lead to under treatment of acute pain and may risk prolonging the hospitalization.

How to Taper Opioids for Acute on Chronic Non-cancer Pain

Unfortunately, there have been no controlled trials to determine optimal tapering of opioids for acute on chronic non-cancer pain. There is also little data to guide weaning of opioids for outpatients with chronic non-cancer pain without any acute pain. Despite these shortcomings, many groups and societies have released opioid tapering guidelines for patients with chronic non-cancer pain [8–12], and we encourage the reader to review these. Debate surrounds the merits of rapid (<1 week) versus slow tapers [13], and thus rapidity of the process should be left to clinician judgement. As one reference states, "finding a plan that an individual patient can embrace with a significant degree of personal engagement might be more important than following a specific protocol" [13].

There is literature to support opioid rotation with buprenorphine or methadone to facilitate tapering of opioids for chronic non-cancer pain [13]. However, as we are only addressing the tapering of opioids for acute on chronic non-cancer pain, we do not advise rotation to buprenorphine or methadone for this purpose. These opioids have unique pharmacological properties that makes medication rotation challenging. In our experience, we have found it easier to simply taper patients to their baseline opioid levels using the same oral opioid they received as inpatients, thus avoiding any medication rotation. For example, if a patient was on 60 mg of oxycodone daily for chronic non-cancer pain, and was escalated to a total of 100 mg oxycodone daily as an inpatient to treat acute pain, we advise tapering to baseline opioid levels using oxycodone rather than rotation to a different opioid. When tapering, we have found it easier to first reduce the dose given at each time rather than reducing the dose frequency, although there is no data to support one method over the other [13]. For example, a patient taking 10 mg oxycodone QID who is being tapered by 50% should be changed to 5 mg QID rather than 10 mg BID.

A review of opioid tapering for chronic non-cancer pain by Berna et al states that opioid doses can be reduced by as much as 75% each day (e.g., 100 mg of morphine on day 1 can be reduced to 25 mg on day 2) and withdrawal is not likely to occur [13]. We have found such a reduction to be too aggressive for patients recovering from acute on chronic non-cancer pain, and thus recommend a more gradual taper (Table 45.1). While tapering opioids as an outpatient for acute on chronic pain, we recommend weekly or biweekly clinic visits until the patient is back to their baseline opioid regimen.

Consequences of Opioid Tapering

Withdrawal

When trying to taper patients with acute on chronic non-cancer pain back to their baseline opioid regimen, one of the goals is to avoid opioid withdrawal. Although withdrawal symptoms can usually be avoided, even with a rapid taper, clinicians should still monitor patients for symptoms and treat appropriately; Table 45.2 lists common symptoms and treatments [14].

These symptoms can more formally be detected using various scales, included the Clinical Opiate Withdrawal Scale or Subjective Opiate Withdrawal Scale [13]. Symptoms can appear two to three half-lives after the last received opioid dose, and thus may appear as early as a few hours depending on the opioid [13, 15] (Table 45.3). Peak symptoms and duration is also dependent on the type of opioid (Table 45.3). Withdrawal is rarely life threatening [13, 14], although there are case reports of death due to dehydration from vomiting and diarrhea [16]. The excess sympathetic activity seen with opioid withdrawal can rarely cause left ventricular dysfunction and subsequent acute heart failure, underscoring the benefits of sympatholytics (e.g., clonidine) for treatment of withdrawal [17, 18].

Worsening Pain

If opioids are tapered before acute on chronic pain starts to resolve, acute pain is likely to worsen. Some patients fear that tapering opioids to baseline levels after acute pain resolves could worsen their chronic pain. However, this concern may be

Table 45.2 Opioid withdrawal symptoms and possible treatments

Symptom	Possible treatment
Aches, myalgias, cramps	NSAIDs, acetaminophen
Diarrhea	Loperamide
Nausea/vomiting	Ondansetron, promethazine, metoclopramide
Insomnia	Trazodone
Anxiety, irritability, rhinorrhea, lacrimation	Hydroxyzine, quetiapine
Autonomic symptoms (HTN, tachycardia, diaphoresis)	Clonidine

Modified from Kral [14]

Table 45.3 Time course of opioid withdrawal after last dose [15]

Opioid	Onset (h)	Peak intensity	Duration
Morphine, oxycodone	6–18	36–72 h	7–10 days
Fentanyl	2–6	6–12 h	4–5 days
Methadone	24–48	3–21 days	6–7 weeks

Modified from Mitra [15]

overstated and patients should be reassured [13]. Interestingly, when patients with chronic non-cancer pain undergo opioid tapers, they often report longer-term improvement in function and decreases in their chronic pain [13].

Conclusions

- Given the risks of high-dose opioids, clinicians should try to minimize dose escalations when opioid dependent patients are admitted with acute pain, and should make every effort to taper these doses to baseline levels once acute pain subsides.
- No formal trials have been performed to determine optimal tapering schedules of opioids for acute on chronic non-cancer pain. Our recommendations are listed in Table 45.1.
- There are no trials comparing the outcomes of fast (<1 week) versus slower opioid tapers, and thus the speed of the taper should be left to clinician judgement.
- If opioids are tapered before acute on chronic pain starts to resolve, acute pain is likely to worsen.
- Patients should be monitored for withdrawal symptoms during an opioid taper and treated with adjunct therapies to control symptoms if needed. Withdrawal is rarely life-threatening, although case reports of death and cardiac morbidity have been reported.

References

1. Hooten WM, Mantilla CB, Sandroni P, Townsend CO. Associations between heat pain perception and opioid dose among patients with chronic pain undergoing opioid tapering. Pain Med. 2010;11(11):1587–98.
2. Chu LF, D'Arcy N, Brady C, Zamora AK, Young CA, Kim JE, et al. Analgesic tolerance without demonstrable opioid-induced hyperalgesia: a double-blinded, randomized, placebo-controlled trial of sustained-release morphine for treatment of chronic nonradicular low-back pain. Pain. 2012;153(8):1583–92.
3. Lewis NL, Williams JE. Acute pain management in patients receiving opioids for chronic and cancer pain. Pain. 2005;5(4):127–9.
4. Chapman CR, Davis J, Donaldson GW, Naylor J, Winchester D. Postoperative pain trajectories in chronic pain patients undergoing surgery: the effects of chronic opioid pharmacotherapy on acute pain. J Pain. 2011;12(12):1240–6.
5. Huxtable CA, Roberts LJ, Somogyi AA, MacIntyre PE. Acute pain management in opioid-tolerant patients: a growing challenge. Anaesth Intensive Care. 2011;39(5):804–23.
6. Patanwala AE, Jarzyna DL, Miller MD, Erstad BL. Comparison of opioid requirements and analgesic response in opioid-tolerant versus opioid-naive patients after total knee arthroplasty. Pharmacotherapy. 2008;28(12):1453–60.
7. Dowell D, Haegerich TM, Chou R. CDC guideline for prescribing opioids for chronic pain - United States, 2016. MMWR Recomm Rep. 2016;65(1):1–49.
8. Chou R, Fanciullo GJ, Fine PG, Adler JA, Ballantyne JC, Davies P, et al. Clinical guidelines for the use of chronic opioid therapy in chronic noncancer pain. J Pain. 2009;10(2):113–30.

9. Manchikanti L, Abdi S, Atluri S, Balog CC, Benyamin RM, Boswell MV, et al. American Society of Interventional Pain Physicians (ASIPP) guidelines for responsible opioid prescribing in chronic non-cancer pain: part 2-guidance. Pain Physician. 2012;15(3):67–116.
10. Affairs DoV. VA/DoD clinical practice guideline for management of opioid therapy for chronic pain. 2010.
11. Kahan M, Mailis-Gagnon A, Wilson L, Srivastava A. Canadian guideline for safe and effective use of opioids for chronic noncancer pain: clinical summary for family physicians. Part 1: general population. Can Fam Physician. 2011;57(11):1257–66.
12. Group WAMD. Interagency guideline on opioid dosing for chronic noncancer pain. 2010.
13. Berna C, Kulich RJ, Rathmell JP. Tapering long-term opioid therapy in chronic noncancer pain: evidence and recommendations for everyday practice. Mayo Clin Proc. 2015;90(6):828–42.
14. Kral LA, Jackson K, Uritsky TJ. A practical guide to tapering opioids. Mental Health Clin. 2015;5(3):102–8.
15. Mitra S, Sinatra RS. Perioperative management of acute pain in the opioid-dependent patient. Anesthesiology. 2004;101(1):212–27.
16. Darke S, Larney S, Farrell M. Yes, people can die from opiate withdrawal. Addiction. 2016;112(2):199–200.
17. Spadotto V, Zorzi A, Elmaghawry M, Meggiolaro M, Pittoni GM. Heart failure due to 'stress cardiomyopathy': a severe manifestation of the opioid withdrawal syndrome. Eur Heart J Acute Cardiovasc Care. 2013;2(1):84–7.
18. Rivera JM, Locketz AJ, Fritz KD, Horlocker TT, Lewallen DG, Prasad A, et al. "Broken heart syndrome" after separation (from OxyContin). Mayo Clin Proc. 2006;81(6):825–8.

Index

© Springer Nature Switzerland AG 2022
D. A. Edwards et al. (eds.), *Hospitalized Chronic Pain Patient*,
https://doi.org/10.1007/978-3-031-08376-1

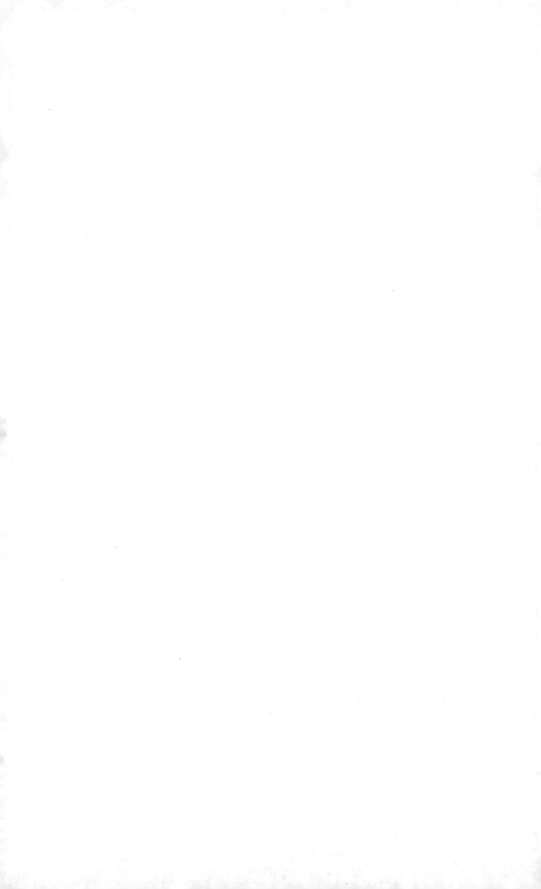

Printed in the United States
by Baker & Taylor Publisher Services